Surger ~~ ..u

Surgery and Beyond

Frank J. Lepreau, M.D.

Old Harbor Publishing
Westport, MA 02790

Please direct correspondence and book orders to:
Frank J. Lepreau, M.D.
74 Old Harbor Road
Westport, MA 02790

ISBN: 0-9766-9370-4

Printed by AlphaGraphics, New Bedford MA

In memory of my wife, Miriam Barwood Lepreau,
and for our children,
Lucy Ann, Judy, Sue, Jay and Mimi,
who shared her limitless love.

"Searching from memory might be compared to throwing the beam of a strong light from your hilltop campsite back over the road you traveled by day. Only a few of the objects you passed are clearly illuminated . . . but memory has advantages that compensate for its failings. By eliminating detail, it clarifies the picture as a whole. Like an artist's brush, it finds higher value in life's essence than in its photographic intricacy."

Charles H. Lindbergh, <u>The Spirit of St. Louis,</u>
Charles Scribner and Sons, 1953

Table of Contents

Surgery and Beyond

Acknowledgements

Viola Pettey Gay has been my helpmeet from the beginning. She has been patient, supportive and diligent in pursuing so many details without which this memoir would not have been possible. Paula Byron and her staff at Harvard Medical Alumni Bulletin have given me many helpful suggestions. Anna Ratcliffe was my earliest typist. James Howard advised on the first chapters. Margo Monahan checked the final manuscript.

Introduction

This was prepared for my 70th Dartmouth College class reunion held in October 2004.

My education as a physician began on a cold February day in 1934 when Bob Michelet was taken out of Dick's House and I was taken in with the same untreatable pneumonia that killed him. Fortunately I had a wise physician whose only therapy was his own comforting presence and wide open windows on the three sides of my room. All 24 hours of each worrisome day, I looked forward to my doctor's visit. While holding my hand, he was reassuring me, but also assessing my condition: my pulse – was it weak, thin, irregular, rapid, too fast or too slow? Was my charted temperature of 104° really accurate? He observed the nuances of my breathing. Were my nostrils flaring as they searched for air? I learned what it was like to be mortally ill and learned that the small bedside observations of a caring physician could be so important.

During my four years in medical school, except for the single month I went home, I was totally immersed in learning from inspiring teachers who were not always gentle. I still remember their exhortations, especially the time I stood at the operating table and repeatedly passed the wrong instruments to the professor. He looked at me

Introduction

and barked, "What's your name?" "Lepreau," I said. "Lepreau, if you want to be a surgeon you will have to learn to make up your mind." That was sixty some years ago, and I still hear the words.

On another day the professor of urology, Dr. Quinby, an intimidating figure, was hosting his East Coast peers. I stood alone in the old Peter Bent Brigham amphitheater presenting my case with the VIP's and my classmates looking down at me. Again, that awesome question, "What's your name?" "Lepreau." "Lepreau, that's muddy thinking. Sit down."

One day, four of us, probably including my roommate, Emerson Day '34, were with Sam Levine. We asked him to name one characteristic, just one, that he felt was essential for a good physician. "Generosity" was his immediate reply.

Upon graduation, I did not get the coveted internship at the Brigham, and I felt that disaster had struck. I called on Howard Clute '11, a distinguished Boston surgeon, who called on a friend, Jay Gile '16, chief surgeon at the Mary Hitchcock Hospital. Within a week I had a 12-month appointment in pathology, an attic room in the home of Dr. Ralph Miller '24, meals at the hospital and a bicycle to get there. The Dartmouth connection not only rescued my professional career but also introduced me to the smartest and most beautiful girl in the world. Miriam Barwood had been valedictorian at the Hanover High School, graduated from Wellesley College, and was there at Mary Hitchcock when I showed up. She became my wife.

Monny and I were married in 1939 and left Mary Hitchcock soon afterward for New Haven and Yale. After five years I became the resident surgeon. Hearing of the Hartford Circus fire, some of us went there to treat burn patients and received considerable experience in skin grafting.

At the behest of a classmate, Paul Magnuson '34, I went into private practice in New Bedford, Massachusetts, but solo practice did not appeal. I accepted a position as assistant to Warren Atwood '15, at the Truesdale Clinic in Fall River. There I practiced general and thoracic surgery and became a busy and successful surgeon. We settled in as a family in nearby Westport where I did my duty in community affairs – public and private school committees, cleaning up the Westport River, passing the first zoning laws. It is good for a physician to hold a minor elective office. It cuts you down to size. No longer in your authoritative long white coat, you are just another guy like the garbage collector sitting next to you.

At some time in the early 1950's I made my first vacation and medical trip overseas to Grand Cayman. The Caymans had not been "discovered." Electricity was available four hours a day for the dentists' drill. There was no refrigeration. We went to the dock to get fresh turtle meat and brought it home on a string dangling from the handlebars of the bicycle. I did an appendectomy on a 19-year-old woman using some old instruments found in a dusty carton. The judicial system was such a contrast to the segregated USA. I saw a black judge officiating at a trial where a white solicitor general was arguing his case in front of a pepper and salt jury.

At the age of 50, while I still had the skill and my health, I acted on my life-long dream of becoming a medical missionary. I first went to the Society of Friends' primitive hospital in rural Kenya for two months with my wife and two small children. I did not mind the paucity of sophisticated equipment – I rather enjoyed it. My eight years of post-graduate training and a long period as a general and thoracic surgeon made me confident that I could handle almost anything surgical. And I did, sometimes with a book beside me, and once commandeering a skeleton. But the mores of an old time mission station were too restrictive for us.

So in 1964, I signed on at the Hôpital Albert Schweitzer, a modern 133-bed hospital in the middle of rural Haiti. Funded by Dr. W. L. Mellon of the Pittsburgh family, the hospital was looking for a person with my training. No private patients. Each visit cost 40 cents and could provide immunization shots or surgery for the removal of a tubercular lung. Haiti turned out to be "just what the doctor ordered" for my wife, our two youngest children and me. We had 10 physicians, a long stream of very sick patients and good equipment and drugs to care for them. If you liked doctoring and operating, this was heaven. No lawyers, no insurance forms, just an unending stream of sick asking for help.

In Haiti I found that tetanus was a major problem. The work we did on tetanus popularized diazepam as the best single medication for treating tetanus patients and made superior bedside nursing care a must. Our results were reported in The Lancet: 985 consecutive cases, excluding newborn, with a mortality of 22%. For newborns our mortality dropped to 26% - the best in the world.

While there I maintained a rotation of resident physicians from Cincinnati and initiated an arrangement with Vermont, Yale, public health people from Harvard, and pediatricians from Tufts. They came for 3 to 4 months and it was great. We were so isolated in that tortured land and yet were on the end of a pipeline of medical people from Mecca, among them David Crombie '59 and Stephen Stein '64. I gave the Yale surgical residents as much operating experience as they could handle while I worked just down the hall to keep them out of trouble. We had a great colleagueship – all learning together. I took a one-month hiatus to Newfoundland and Labrador, exchanging places with Dr. Gordon Thomas of the Grenfell Mission.

After returning to the United States I had a major re-entry problem. I fled to Appalachia and the Frontier Nursing Service in Hyden, Kentucky, population 400. The service trained nurse midwives, and treated coal miners and their families. I learned much about living conditions there and about John L. Lewis and his drive for portal-to-portal pay. I descended four times into the mines, a half-mile or so, which was not so dangerous as it sounds in a well run mine. Black lung resulting from the soft coal mined in Kentucky was not a debilitating malady. Cigarettes were the real villains.

After two years we returned to Westport where I functioned as a general practitioner. I became active in the Brown University Medical School, which sent me for a week to the island of Leyte in the Philippines to appraise a community-based medical school. While there I stood on Red Beach where two of my contemporaries – GI's – had waded ashore under fire. On another occasion I went to St. Lucia, in the Caribbean to see if Brown could send students there. The Brown connection was fun since I always had a student with me.

I was active in the Massachusetts Medical Society, especially with a small committee of colleagues who befriended other society members who had drug, social, or alcohol problems. That project was a great success. In Fall River, a businessman, a psychiatric social worker, and I started a public treatment center for alcoholics and drug addicts. For 25 years I treated them all, including pregnant addicts. The program has burgeoned because of the dedicated staff. My final professional endeavor was as a physician for terminally ill cancer patients at the Rose Hawthorne Home in Fall River. I saw my last patient there in 2002 on August 15th.

I lost my wife, Monny, in 1994. Together we had five children; four are still alive. My three daughters have careers in nursing, histology and counseling. My son is in academia.

Beginning with Dr. Harry French '13 in Dick's House, Dartmouth has been a major help along my way, right up to recent years when Tim Flanigan '79 taught me how to treat AIDS. It's been a great ride. Now 70 years out, the road gets a little bumpy.

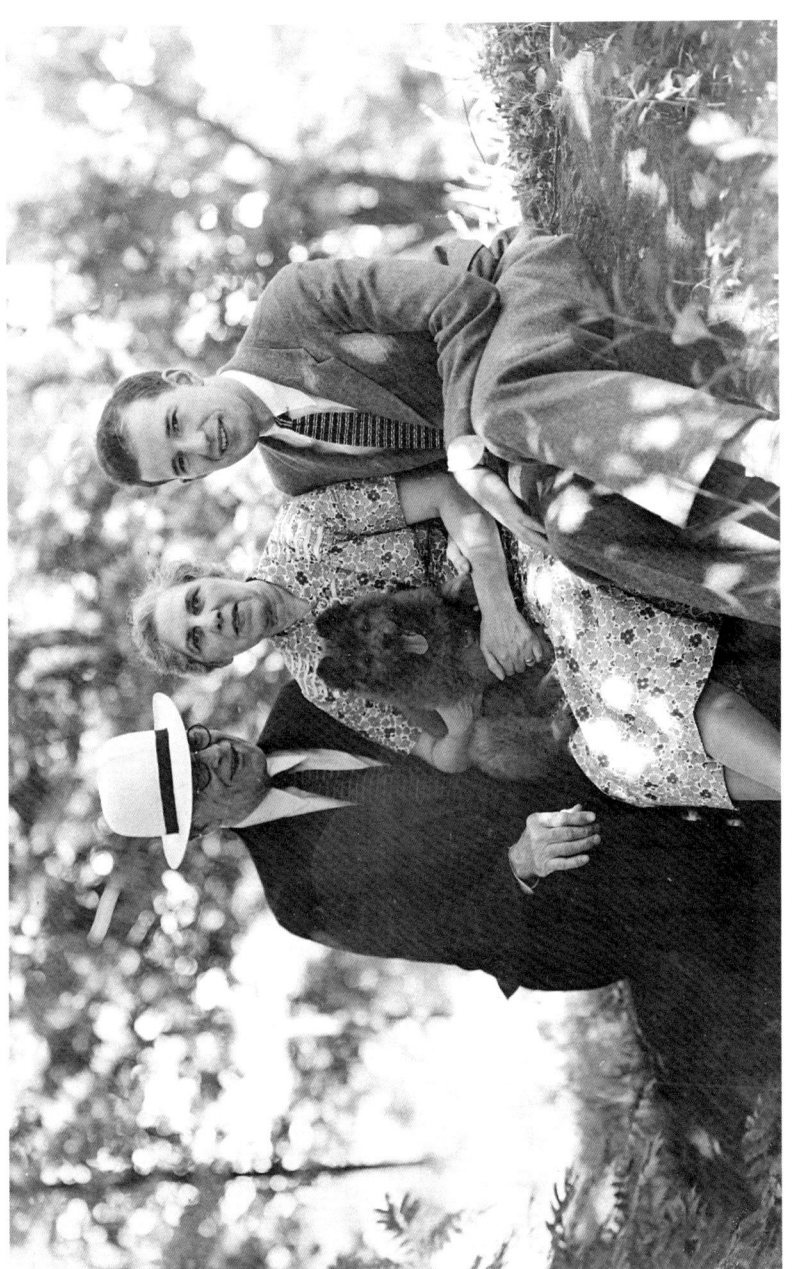

Family – Hastings-on-Hudson, NY - 1934

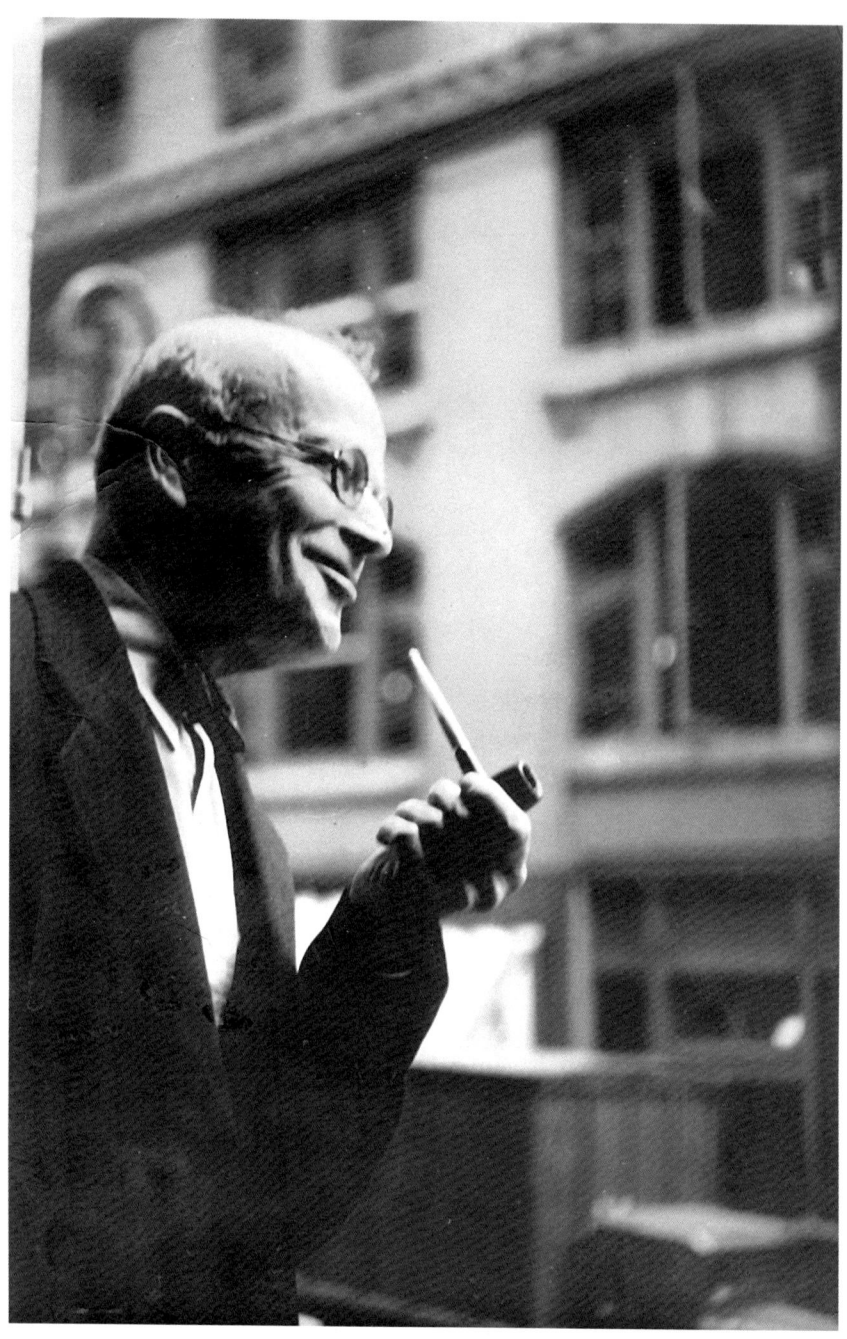

My Father

1

Early Years

My father was a Frenchman, born in 1875 in the modest sized town of Laon in the north of France. Laon had been overrun by the Germans in the Franco-Prussian War and was destroyed again in WWI and yet again in WWII. My father was one of thirteen children, six sons and seven daughters. Once a week, he told me, all the boys gathered in the courtyard and showered together with my grandfather. The girls did the same with my grandmother. By decree of the *pater familias* a military career loomed in my father's future and in 1893 he was enrolled in St. Cyr, the French equivalent of West Point. But after a year of slogging through the jungles of French Africa, he wanted out. The response was, "You are on your own."

So at the age of nineteen he came alone through Ellis Island with nothing more than his duffel, a few francs, and a lot of drive. Making the most of his French accent, he landed a first job as a croupier at roulette tables in New York City. He moved from place to place, each time climbing a bit higher on the socioeconomic ladder of his newly adopted land. Eventually his ambition carried him to the position of senior vice president and general sales manager for the Thomas A. Edison Company. Few would have guessed that this polished executive helping to preside over one of

America's largest corporations had arrived in this country as a poor young immigrant.

My father married my mother, Marion Amelia Thornton, on November 24, 1897, three years after moving to the United States. In their wedding photo, a strikingly beautiful bride stands alongside a handsome groom with a short, neatly trimmed beard. My mother came from a middle class Chicago family but she rarely talked about them, and consequently I never learned much about her relatives.

My older brother, William Neville Lepreau, was born in 1900. He went away to school in Canada, and then entered the United States Marine Corp in 1917 while still a teenager. He saw combat in World War I and was wounded at two brutal Marine engagements, Belleau Wood and Chateau Thierry. He suffered from shell shock and spent eighteen months in St. Elizabeth's Mental Hospital in Washington, D.C.

I was born on October 6, 1912, at home at 312 South Grove Avenue, Oak Park, Illinois, an upscale area on the west side of Chicago. In later years my mother would tell stories about the marital infidelities of our prestigious neighbors, Ernest Hemingway and Frank Lloyd Wright.

Although she didn't talk much about her family, my mother did have contact with her sister, Irene. Aunt Irene, Uncle Fred Miller, and their son, Freddie, lived in Austin, on the west side of Chicago. Freddie died young, perhaps in his forties, of a heart attack. Uncle Fred worked for the *Chicago Tribune*. Occasionally he would call me and offer, "Hey, Jim! Do you want to go see where so and so got it last night?" "So-and-so" was always some prominent gangster of the day. I'd reply,

"Yes, sure!" And we would get together and visit the area where a mobster had been assassinated the night before. The bloodstains would be visible on the sidewalk and bullet holes peppered nearby brick walls. I thought those experiences were special since they gave me brownie points when I bragged to friends that I'd seen where a thug had "got it" the night before.

I think these were balmy days in Chicago when my father was making it up the corporate ladder in the years before the 1921 financial recession — days of sterling silver, fancy china and custom-made suits. He was employed by Edison to market his new storage battery, which was used in the growing railroad market to activate right-of-way signals. He was successful. I don't suppose my father was close to Edison but I do know he photographed him. He gave me a photograph of Edison he had taken and printed on large paper, which I have given to my grandson, Evan Jose. Dad said he watched when Edison auditioned singers for his records. The singer would be performing in one room. The entire opening into the next room where Edison sat consisted of a big horn, which became progressively smaller until it reached an end piece that fit into Edison's ear.

When he wasn't immersed in his professional life, Dad enthusiastically pursued other aspects of his adopted American culture. He became a Christian Scientist, a religion that I, too, embraced all through my college years. He played golf, managed a railroad baseball team, and belonged to the Chicago Masons and the Shriners. His office was in The People's Gas Building on Michigan Avenue in Chicago, alongside those of railroad men. He traveled frequently and took first-class accommodations. He dressed well and carried a cane. With his French accent, he must have been a charmer.

He was proud of his adopted country but never forgot his French roots. When I was six years old, I recall my parents celebrating the Armistice of World War I on the evening of November 11, 1918 in the dining room of a fancy nightclub or hotel in Washington, D.C. My father stood me up on the table and led the entire room singing the *Marseillaise*, somewhat like Victor Laszlo in *Casablanca* leading the crowd to drown out the Germans in Rick's Café. There are certain people who qualify as good guys; in some indefinable way, my father was one of them.

When we lived in the New York area I recall watching my father walk down the red carpet to the tracks in the Grand Central Station to catch the 20th Century Limited on his way to Chicago. The Century was the New York Central's "crack train," as they called it. It went by the water level route in sixteen hours to Chicago via Albany, Buffalo, Cleveland and "all points west," as Rudy Vallee used to sing. The competition was the Pennsylvania Railroad's similar elite train called *The Broadway Limited*, which went west through the Delaware water gap to Chicago in sixteen hours. The trains left around six in the evening, arriving in Chicago the next morning.

I recall riding in a small elevator in the prestigious Blackstone Hotel on Michigan Avenue in Chicago where my father had taken me to lunch at a restaurant on the roof overlooking the lake. The elevator was activated by pulling on a wire rope which pulled counter weights sequestered somewhere below. That experience at the Blackstone convinced me that my father was important, and he remained so to me forever. Small incidents drew me to him. I recall a mystery game we carried on. I searched for the source of the special flavor that sometimes appeared in my morning oatmeal. It turned out to be only cinnamon, but the search was exciting.

I don't know what inspired Dad, in 1913, to purchase a 200-acre dairy farm in Fairfax County, Virginia. My guess is that he entertained visions of becoming a gentleman farmer. The milk house and barn were the first farm buildings in the United States wired under the Rural Electrification Act. He used Delaval milking machines. Our milk had the highest butter fat percentage and was considered the best around.

I loved the farm. I made and baited small wooden boxes as rabbit traps. One day, while cutting greens for the rabbits, I sliced a fingertip almost off and then reattached it. I still have a scar on my left thumb. We had a horse named Jack to pull the buggy and for riding. I liked to ride Jack early in the day when he was not needed for work. One time in the morning mist, I was the first to see a particular cow calve. I sped back to the house on horseback as if I were carrying the news from Aix to Ghent. I felt so important.

In the summer I walked barefoot a quarter mile up to the mailbox on the Leesburg Pike. It was fun to squeeze the dry dust of our lane between my toes. Near the mailbox there stood a big persimmon tree. I sat underneath it, eating the fruit when it was ripe, soft and tasty.

I was flattered when DeChauney, the French farm manager, let me get up into the silo to stomp down the ensilage as it was blown in at the top. In spite of being a skinny six-year-old, I was certain that I was making a significant contribution. These were Prohibition years and the juice from the ensilage that settled at the bottom of the silo caught the attention of the hands who worked the farm. They devised clever ways of drawing off this alcoholic beverage. My mother, an ardent Women's Christian Temperance Union member, found their cache and caused a furor when, without warning, she poured gallons of it out onto the ground. I've always wondered if her father, who was never mentioned in our household, had been an alcoholic. That might explain her temperance zeal.

Our house at the farm had gutters designed to empty into a rain barrel at one corner to provide "soft" water for laundry. Saturday night we each took a ritual bath in a large round galvanized washtub. This was no problem in warm weather when the bath was carried on outside. But northern Virginia winters can be cold, so during those months the bath was set up in front of a large pot-bellied wood stove. The bath itself wasn't too bad, but the test of fortitude came when I had to dash through the rest of the cold house and upstairs to slide between cold sheets.

As a young child I had my chores to perform. Before we were electrified I spent a lot of time cleaning the soot from the inside of the glass kerosene lamp chimneys. I also collected eggs from the hen house. When it came time for a sacrifice we'd take a chicken to the woodshed and there either chop off its head with a hatchet or wring it around by the head until the neck was broken. Either way the bird was flung on the woodpile to flop around until motionless.

We usually traveled the five miles to Herndon, the nearest town, in a buggy pulled by Jack. He also took us to the Christian Science Church in Falls Church,

Virginia, fifteen miles away. Eventually we bought a Ford touring car. On rare occasions we went to Washington, D.C. in "the machine" as people called an automobile in those days. This meant arising before dawn, storing containers of gasoline and water on the running board, packing materials to patch the tires which were certain to be punctured on the round trip of 50 miles, and bringing plenty of food. To me it seemed like a trip into the great unknown.

One day we were returning in the machine from Washington to Herndon on the Leesburg Pike, now Route 7, which was an elevated gravel road with deep ditches on both sides. We saw a horse and buggy approaching so we slowed down. The horse reared up, screamed and hurled himself and the buggy with its passengers into the ditch. No one was hurt. On one of these visits to Washington, when I was seven years old, I rolled Easter eggs down the White House lawn. It must have been 1919.

One popular hangout for Herndon's 900 inhabitants was a drug store with large colored glass vials in the window. The soda fountain was on the right, just inside the door. We ordered ice cream sodas, which we drank while sitting on the kind of hard-bottom wire-back chairs seen in vintage Coca Cola ads. There was also a general store in town and a railroad station, which was part of the Washington and Old Dominion Railroad. This was a Toonerville Trolley like affair, with one car originating in Rosalyn, Virginia, just outside of Washington and terminating in Bluemont, Virginia.

I lasted exactly one day in the Herndon Public Schools. I was a northerner. The other students harassed and ostracized me. When someone from the farm came to pick me up, they found a lonesome, forlorn and tearful waif. Fortunately my mother soon enrolled me in the welcoming and supportive Herndon Seminary, a one-room school conducted in the home of the Castlemans, four maiden ladies of the Confederacy. As many have told me since, the best teachers should be in the early grades and I had them. Miss Ida and Miss Lulu taught academics, Miss Virginia taught music and Miss Mary made lunch and kept house. In case of bad weather I could stay overnight. Punishment was quick, physical and non-negotiable. Miss Lulu bent my fingers back and rapped my palms with a wooden ruler. The teacher's desk was on a platform and on the wall behind it was a huge Confederate flag. At least one of their relatives had served in the Civil War.

The education was both moral and intellectual. What a way to start in life, living on a working farm and attending the early grades under the care of the genteel Misses Castleman! In my adult life, I served for many years on a public school committee. As a result of my positive early school experience, I have always pushed for the recognition of early elementary school teachers by financial or prestigious rewards.

One of Herndon's main attractions was the Buell family. Mr. Buell was a southern gentleman, a realtor who handled the purchase and eventual sale of our farm. Mrs. Buell was a gracious lady and my mother's friend. The Buells had several daughters, including Alice, with whom I went to kindergarten. I used to look forward to visiting the Buells where we played croquet on their front lawn.

When Bill returned home from St. Elizabeth's Mental Hospital in Washington, my parents did not realize the depth of his mental turmoil resulting from his experiences in World War I. Bill was smart and honest, and he adored our father. He tried his best to work the farm although he knew nothing about farming. I do not know which parent was responsible, but either Mom or Dad was unsympathetic with his ways, and so Bill left. Not long after, in 1921 when I was almost ten, we sold the farm during the recession that cost my father his job with Edison.

After we left the farm, we went to live with old friends in the country near West Nyack, New York. There I made a crystal set radio. It was a skeleton contrivance that used a wire fence as an antenna. One of the components was a Quaker Oats container around which I wound copper wire to make a coil. With earphones I could pick up a barely audible sound, probably from New York City thirty miles away.

Next we moved to a small rental house in West Nyack. These were unhappy years because of severe arguments between my parents and much housework for me - cleaning, cooking, and shopping. It was in that difficult period that I had my nose broken and lost a tooth. I suffered the broken nose in a fistfight with another boy who pulled my stocking cap down on my face, whacked me and was out of sight by the time I recovered. The broken tooth resulted from a fall in a dairy barn.

After I completed the sixth and seventh grades in the West Nyack public schools, we moved to a new house in Hastings-on-the-Hudson, New York. Hastings had three different social groups. One, mostly made up of Hungarians and Poles, was concentrated on the Hudson River near the Anaconda Copper Company. A second group consisted of the more affluent people whose children attended private schools. The third was perched up on a hill. It was a middle class neighborhood called Hudson Heights and was where my family lived.

The eighth and ninth grades in the Hastings schools are a dim memory. I vaguely remember having hot cocoa in the winter in a closed-in porch of an old residence, which served as a schoolhouse. Polly Van Nostrand was a strict but fair teacher. When I talked too much she went behind me and put her fingers into my supraclavicular spaces and shook me hard.

In the early months in Hastings I recall being picked on by some of the boys at school whose fathers worked in the copper mills. They were a tough bunch and they had concluded that I was a sissy. One day as we stood at the blackboard I gave one of them a punch, which must have been effective, for there was no more trouble. Another classmate, Henry Kulakowski, appointed himself my personal defender. He went on to a career as the Masked Marvel of professional wrestling.

A fellow student, Jeannette, was the light of my young life. We passed notes back and forth in school and I walked down to her house singing "Ramona" and "Always." She was a well-formed brunette, accomplished in tennis, swimming, and diving. Her father, Doc Reynolds, was a physical education instructor in a large New York City public high school. At home his energies were devoted to his children and those of the neighborhood; he taught us swimming, diving, tennis, and target shooting with the standard match rifle of the National Rifle Association.

In the winter Doc Reynolds taught us hockey. He piled us into his old air-cooled Franklin sedan, never minding that the skates tore up the upholstery or that the hockey sticks which lay outside in the cleft between the hood and the fenders scratched the paint. Off we went wherever there was ice, usually a pond on an estate where the guardian tried to chase us off. It didn't work. Doc, our hero, with us marshaled behind him, confronted the enemy with a fiery speech along the lines of "Just what harm are these boys doing to your ice?" followed by a barrage about keeping kids out of trouble.

Doc was a fierce competitor. In later years, when we came home from college we thought we could beat him at tennis. No way! Despite his age he countered with short, well-placed chop shots. We loved him. He was a superb example of what a concerned adult can do for children.

The Hastings-on-Hudson years also witnessed the most traumatic episode of my childhood — the death of my Airedale, Rags, poisoned by neighbors who disliked him. I still see him lying dead at the foot of the outside stairs on an autumn morning. I cried and cried. Then I buried him under the grape arbor and placed flowers on his grave. I had other dogs but never one that replaced Rags. In some way this loss of Rags in my childhood was nearly as distressing as the death of my wife decades later.

My parents took me exploring nearby New York City and all that the city had to offer, especially after Dad opened a photographic studio on East 12th Street. We went to the Broadway musicals of the twenties and thirties: "The Desert Song," "No, No Nannette" and the Ziegfield Follies where I saw, besides the legs, Will Rogers swing his lariat and comment on the day's news. My mother introduced me to Shakespeare through *The*

Merchant of Venice. There were movie serials on Saturday afternoons for ten cents, each episode ending with Ruth Roland about to be thrown off a cliff in an encounter with the villain. The following week she was back on her horse with the villain at the bottom of the canyon.

Occasionally Dad took my mother and me, or sometimes just me, to places plush and others not so plush, usually in lower Manhattan. I first noted the importance of tipping the maitre'd at the main dining room of the Waldorf-Astoria where we had gone to celebrate my parents' anniversary. As we entered, Dad slipped the man five dollars, which was quite a bit in the 1930's. We were immediately escorted to the best table at the Fifth Avenue side of the building.

Various respectable Greenwich Village eateries were among Dad's favorites. One was The Black Cat. Another was on McDougal Alley where he wanted me to try his boyhood tonic, a glass filled with equal parts of water and Chianti – poured from a squat, straw-wrapped bottle – into which a beaten raw egg was added. My mother disapproved, but I had it just the same. The Brevoort Hotel and The Lafayette featured French cuisine where I was introduced to frogs' legs.

Saturdays we walked the lower East Side, which was home to many Jewish and Eastern European immigrants. When we ventured to the West Side, we shopped at the pushcarts lined up one next to another, stretching for blocks beneath the 9th Avenue Elevated. Here one could find anything: melons of all kinds, grapes, bananas, fish swimming in galvanized iron tubs, women's underwear, and sticky fly paper.

It seemed to me that I had to do quite a few domestic chores in those years. In West Nyack my responsibilities had included cooking and cleaning up. In Hastings, the coal furnace required constant attention. I also swept the cellar, sifting the ashes outdoors while singing "Yes, We Have No Bananas" and "Barney Google." I maintained a good-sized yard where I planted and tended a vegetable garden. Weekly I scrubbed the bathroom and kitchen floors. One summer was devoted to painting the house. I shopped in the village downtown about a mile away and pulled the groceries up a long hill in my red wagon. And there were screens and storm windows to put up and take down. When I was older I became a professional storm window repairman for a while because my glazing was so good. I charged top price at the time – 75 cents an hour.

My one hobby as a teenager was photography, one of the pursuits my father developed to keep us solvent in the thirties. We would walk around the neighborhood, take a picture of a residence with the old five-by-seven box camera, develop the film in our bathroom and put the picture in a fancy ten-cent frame. A few days later, looking like a Charles Dickens waif, I usually succeeded in selling it to the owner of the house for a handsome fee.

During my last three years of high school we spent the winters in Glen Ellyn, a suburb of Chicago, then moved back to Hastings in the summer to accommodate my father's job changes. In the depths of the Depression my father would come home day after hot summer day having spent hours pounding the pavements of New York. Unsuccessful in finding a job, he trudged a mile uphill from the Hastings Railroad Station to our house once again. There were millions like him in those sad times. Undaunted, he kept at it. We were always well fed, housed and warm. Dad never complained and remained supportive of my brother during his difficult times.

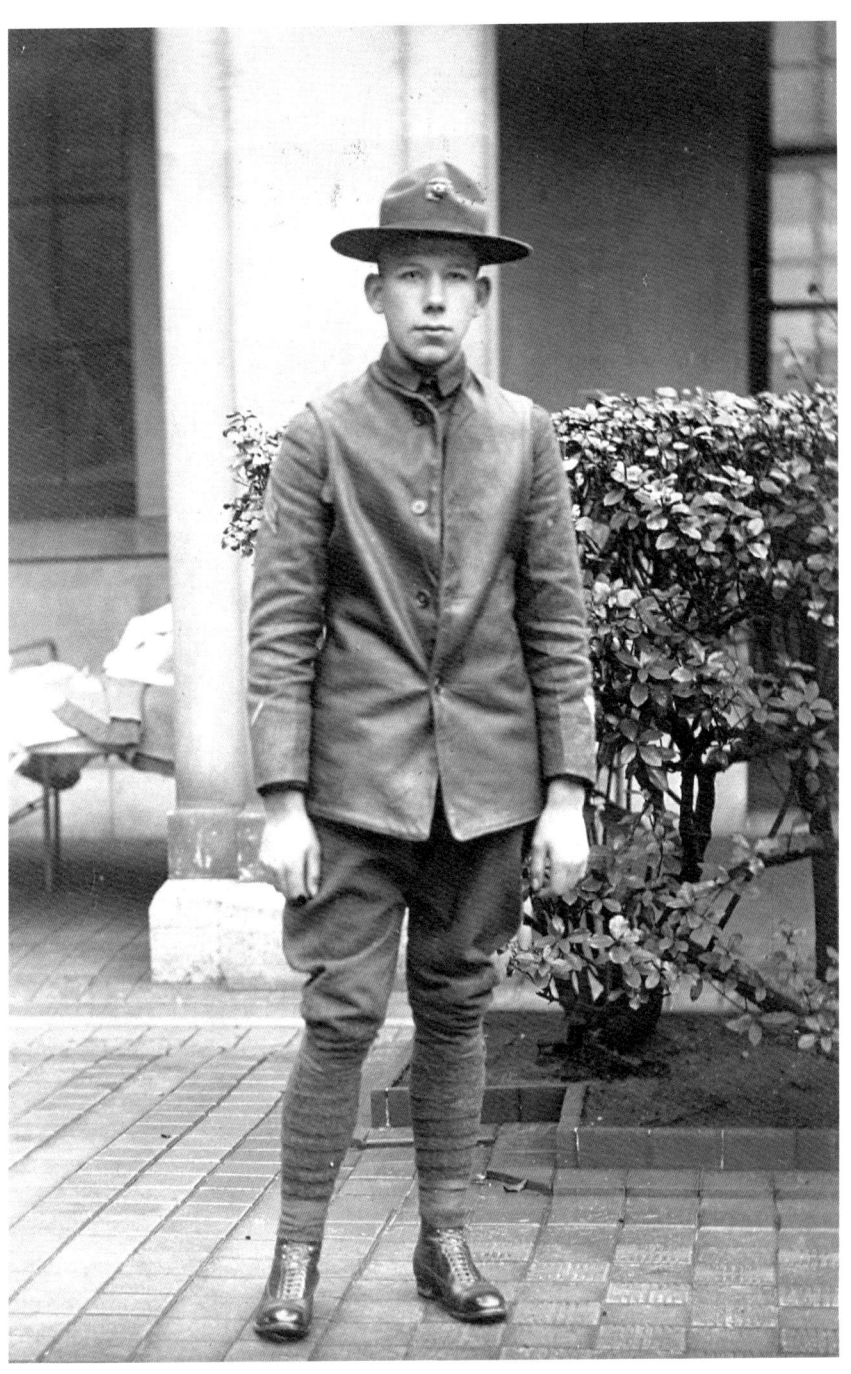

My brother Bill, U.S. Marine - Paris 1919

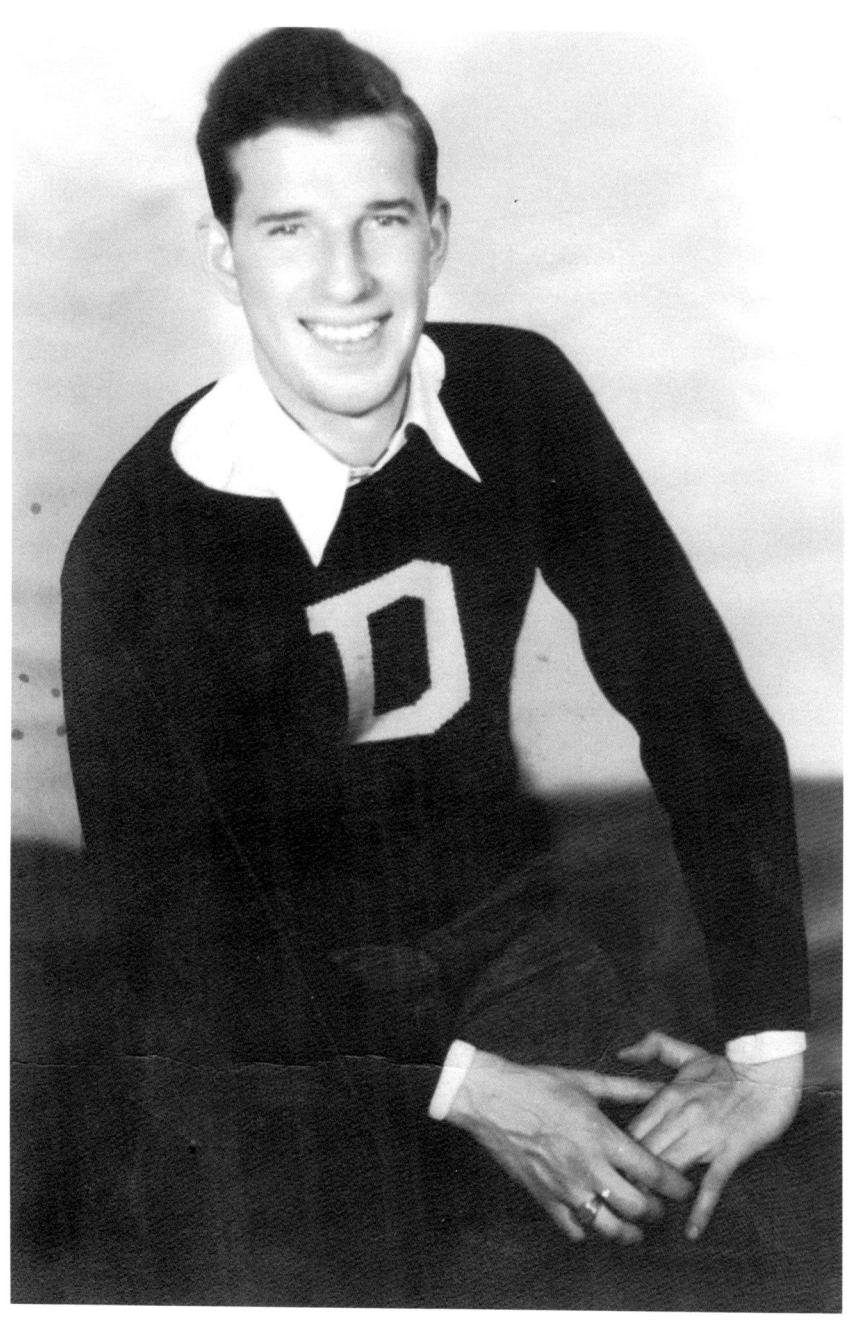

Joe College

2

Dartmouth College – 1930 to 1934

It was during my high school years in Glen Ellyn that I became a so-so athlete running the mile and earning a big "G" emblazoned on my chest. I became a senior patrol leader in the Boy Scouts. I graduated from Glenbard Township High School in 1930 and chose Dartmouth College because of its proximity to the New Hampshire mountains and the Connecticut River and many outdoor activities. My high school friends thought it was snobbery that motivated me to "go east" to school. Not so. It was the Dartmouth Outing Club that drew me.

I was fortunate to be admitted to Dartmouth on certification by my high school because of its academic standing, thus avoiding the usual preadmission examination. It was the fall of 1930, the financial world had collapsed in October 1929, and the country was tobogganing into the Depression. No one seemed to have much money for college and I suppose the applicant pool had shrunk.

Dartmouth tuition in 1930 was $400, the same amount I would pay to Harvard Medical School four years later. My father managed to give me $1,000 the year I entered college and told me that I, myself, should manage the $600 left over after tuition. It was good for my discipline. I supported myself with restaurant jobs and a college loan during the academic year. In the summer, I scraped and painted houses with a blowtorch in one hand and a large putty knife in the other while standing on a ladder. What was I thinking?

I lived in the cheapest dormitory, College Hall, for $150 a year. My college life was not a party. My time was taken up with restaurant jobs, athletics year round, and efforts to stay awake at night to learn something. My grades were fair. I started as a geology major and foolishly switched to chemistry. That was a disaster because I was not smart enough to handle it and the competition was fierce.

College Hall was the home of several athletes from the public schools of Lawrence, Lowell and Somerville, old crumbling mill towns in the suburbs of Boston. One of the athletes, Deac Campbell, extricated me from the dishpan at the local greasy spoon and got me a job waiting tables and washing dishes at the Rood Club. I was amazed to see at the Dartmouth Winter Carnival in February, 1931, at the very depths of the Depression, students breezing into the restaurant at 1:00 a.m. dressed in white tie and tails, escorting gorgeous women clad in ankle-length mink coats. Obviously not everyone had been wiped out in 1929. By the following fall, I had worked my way up to the position of cook. I made mashed potatoes with lots of butter and cream and passed the meals from the stove to the waiters.

During my freshman year in 1930, students spoke with affection and admiration of Nelson Rockefeller, who had just graduated and had worked as a waiter at Mrs. Rood's. Rockefeller was truly a "big man on campus." He belonged to Casque and Gauntlet, a prestigious senior society. He also served in the student governing body and captained the soccer team. The house where he lived was located on the corner of the main intersection in

Hanover. It had an open porch where the students sat observing the world of Hanover, particularly its female residents. My future wife, Monny, who was local, later told me that when she had to pass by the house, she would tighten her buttocks so she wouldn't wobble.

At Dartmouth I made the freshman cross country and track teams, receiving my 1934 numerals in both, which meant I was reasonably good. Subsequently I achieved nine varsity letters. I did well in winter sports on snowshoes because there were not many people crazy enough to do it. The snowshoeing course ran across fields, through trails in the woods, down railroad tracks, and over fences. Our clothing consisted of underpants and a suit of long winter underwear, heavy wool socks, no shoes and a skeleton bit of wool around the head to cover our ears.

The best part of my athletic endeavors consisted of the trips to competitions. In spite of the Depression, there was somehow enough money to put us up at the Statler Hotel in Boston, a rather expensive hotel at the time. There were two trips to the Seignory Club up the Ottawa River from Montreal. The Seignory Club was a resort catering to affluent people from Montreal and Ottawa. On New Year's Eve, we were sumptuously fed and entertained in the company of the glamorous daughter of the premier of Quebec. Canada did not suffer prohibition and it was high life for us students.

At one of our athletic meets in Canada, I won a race making me the North American Snowshoe Champion! There were few competitors but I won the title after competing repeatedly against Andberg, my nemesis from the University of New Hampshire. Jack Shea was among my teammates, that included snowshoers, speed skaters, long distance skaters, figure skaters, ski jumpers, downhill skiers, slalom skiers, and cross country skiers. He later went on to capture two gold medals at the 1932 Olympics held in his hometown of Lake Placid, New York. I experienced a vicarious thrill from wearing Jack's skates to circle the Olympic arena in Lake Placid.

When not competing on snowshoes, I put on my running shoes. Dartmouth had recently installed one of the best indoor wooden tracks in the country. Glenn Cunningham of national fame once set a record on our track. It was exciting coming off a curve in spikes on the wood surface. One year on the boards in the Boston Garden I ran a two-mile race neck and neck with Arthur Pier of Harvard. We exchanged the lead frequently. Seated alongside the straightaway at the finish was my date, Betty French, a Wellesley student, with her father. He was a distinguished Dartmouth alumnus and president of the Boston and Maine Railroad, which owned the Boston Garden. I can't remember who won, but I do remember how exciting it was to hear the crowd yelling. Arthur Pier and I crossed paths many years later. As I had, Arthur went on to Harvard Medical School. He became an esteemed family practitioner making house calls in Boston's elite Beacon Hill area.

In my senior year I was captain of the cross-country team. I don't recall how our team performed but probably not very well. I do remember the agony of the hills on the six-mile run in Van Courtland Park in New York City. I collapsed at the finish and woke up in the locker room vomiting all over the place. My father was beside me. He must have wondered at what price that stupid son of his was seeking glory.

In the summer of 1933 following the completion of our junior year at Dartmouth, a few classmates and I went to Chicago to see the World's Fair. After the fair, I decided to return to Hastings-on-Hudson by train, duplicating the adventures of Harry Espencheid, a friend from Dartmouth. Harry occasionally rode the rails to Canada and, in spite of being a teetotaler, often brought back expensive liquor for fellow students. "For a price, Uguarte, for a price!" as Bogie would say.

I went to the LaSalle Street Station, procured a timetable, and decided that the Lake Shore Limited sounded like a reasonably fast train with some glamour to it, at least in the name. It was scheduled to leave the station in the dark of early evening. The station yards were open so I walked around and over the tracks, avoiding the trains entering and leaving until I found my train. I was dressed in a blue cotton shirt and wool pants with nothing more than one or two dollars in bills sewn into the cuff of my pants and a determination to follow the techniques outlined by my mentor. One must wait patiently until the train starts before mounting and be sure to get off before it stops. Above all, be on the lookout for the ever-present "bulls" or railroad detectives. They were mean. They didn't arrest riders without tickets but would beat them up with clubs. Fortunately, I avoided them my entire trip.

The classic steam engine train makeup began with the engine followed by the tender. The front two thirds of the tender was filled with coal, which was shoveled into the firebox by hand. The last third contained the water tank with an opening on top about five feet in diameter so that water could be taken on from watering tanks on the side of the tracks. Or, to save time, water could be scooped up on the fly from a long trough between the tracks. The next car was usually a baggage car without openings on the ends. The passenger cars, which followed the baggage car, had an accordion-like affair on each end that hooked on to a similar arrangement on adjoining cars to keep passengers out of the weather when they walked from car to car. That was the ideal place to ride, in the accordion facing the blind end of the baggage car, hence the term blind baggage, or "the blinds". One could sit or stand there and be reasonably comfortable, sheltered from the elements.

I found my train, hung around behind switch boxes, waited until it started and jumped on. There I found three other riders, two black men and a young white man, who was intoxicated and carrying a bottle of hard liquor. He made us all nervous, so when the train paused while crossing Michigan, we put him off. Every time the train stopped we all got off, ran, hid in the bushes and waited until it started up again. Only then would we remount.

Detroit was different. My fellow travelers ran hard this time and didn't stop near the train but kept going. Finally I found one of them and said, "What's it all about?" My companions kept me out of trouble by explaining that when the train went across the international bridge into Windsor, Canada it was floodlit. In Windsor, all riders like ourselves were taken off and put on a rock pile. It took exactly thirty days to get enough money to buy a ticket back into the United States.

So in Detroit, I hopped a train to Toledo and rode between two cars hanging on to an iron stepladder. I tied myself on with a belt because I was afraid that I might fall asleep. Once I got to Toledo I made my way to the highways and grabbed a ride on an empty transport truck which had a narrow, flat place designed for the wheels of the automobiles. I lay down in that narrow space and went to sleep untied, a foolish thing to do as I could have easily fallen off.

Near the outskirts of Cleveland Union Station, I learned the station was impenetrable. Although I had only one dollar left, I took a taxi around Cleveland to East Cleveland for ninety cents leaving me ten cents to finance the rest of the trip to Hastings. At East Cleveland the Lake Shore Limited and other eastbound trains changed from electric or diesel engines back to steam. I hid in the bushes at the side of the switching yards and hopped a steam train. With no blind baggage car available, I was forced to ride the whole distance on top of the water tank, a miserable experience because the train didn't stop for water but took it up on the fly from between the tracks. There I was, clad in a thin shirt, clinging to the top of the water tank traveling sixty miles an hour or more through the cold night across New York State. The wind combined with the evaporation from my shirt caused me excessive discomfort. To try to relieve the cold, I did all kinds of stupid things like hanging out over the edge of the tender or getting on top of the first passenger car. The passenger car didn't have an accordion on it so I was lying down on top of it with very little to hold on to. Obviously I survived, but it was a stupid thing to have done.

I stayed on that train into Harmon, New York, which was north of Hastings. Here the trains changed from steam to electric. I don't remember how I came from Harmon to Hastings but I do remember finally walking up to my house and knocking on the door. My father answered but did not recognize me. My mother also failed to recognize me until I started to speak. She then broke down and cried, for I was black, black, black. I had been periodically saturated with water, and all the smoke, dust and ashes from the firebox had stuck to my skin. I had an adventure, yes, but a foolhardy one—one slip and it would have been all over for me.

Following my adventure on America's railways, I returned to Dartmouth. The high point of my college career came during that time and had nothing to do with sports. In response to a midnight knock on my door, I opened it. There stood Red Rolfe, captain of the baseball team and a Big Man on Campus. Rolfe was a modest boy from New Hampshire and he remained that way during a long career as the star third baseman with the Yankees when they were in their prime with players like Lazzeri, Ruth, and Dickey. He had come to ask me to join Sphinx, his senior society, which consisted of a small group of students accomplished in a variety of extracurricular activities. I was ecstatic.

At the urging of my friends, I also joined a fraternity. Even though they voted me president, I never did become the classic fraternity man. I was either too busy or too tired. One of my fraternity brothers was Tom Curtis, a brilliant student, who went on to become a U.S. representative from St. Louis. Years after our graduation from Dartmouth, he took my wife and me to lunch in the House dining room, where he pointed to John Kennedy and speculated that one day Kennedy just might be president of the United States.

One June, I went with a group of friends from the Ledyard Canoe Club on a canoe trip. We put our three canoes into Lake Champlain at Burlington, Vermont, and expected to paddle down to Poughkeepsie, New York, for an intercollegiate rowing competition. The trip was work. The day's routine started with a full, hot breakfast, then sandwiches on the fly and a good meal in a town restaurant in the evening, where we bought the next day's food. One evening when I was carrying the eggs for breakfast, my bag broke and the eggs fell to the sidewalk. Our banker, Harry Espencheid, made me scrape them up. His attitude may have been why we made him the keeper of the purse. The most beautiful scene of the trip was paddling in the moonlight in perfect stillness through Mother's Bunch, a collection of small islands in Lake George. At Albany, paddling fiercely under a bridge, we could barely make progress against the tide. Somewhere down the Hudson we hitched a ride on a barge in order to make the Poughkeepsie regatta.

In some ways, sports and social activities eclipsed academics for me at Dartmouth. My college academic career was average. I majored in chemistry, which was way beyond my intellect. Phi Beta Kappa types, who went on to be VIP's in DuPont and other prestigious corporations, surrounded me. Professor Andrew Scarlett, chief of the Department of Chemistry, had some final words for me, "Lepreau, you'll never graduate from the Harvard Medical School." He had no reason to think otherwise, given my performance in his department. Yet he and his wife were kind to me when I was recovering from pneumonia in the spring of 1934, my senior year at Dartmouth.

During the years before I met my wife, I had several romances. One was with Mary Matychik, an attractive, brilliant student whose Polish mother, a widow, did not care for me. Another was with Peggy Sawyer, a nice young woman whose father worked at the Rockefeller Institute. Years later I learned he was the great Wilbur Sawyer who developed the vaccine for yellow fever. I think it was most likely distance that terminated that affair, as we were shuttling between Glen Ellyn and Hastings.

Gail Hall was another girlfriend. She came to visit me at Dartmouth a few times, once for the Dartmouth Winter Carnival when I suffered a severe ankle sprain. She spent most of the gala weekend in my living quarters keeping my foot in ice water; nothing else happened. She graduated from Wheaton, where I visited a few times while in Boston. Wheaton had courting rooms called Hebe's parlors, small cell-like nooks across which a heavy drapery could be pulled.

I might as well get on with my other pre-marriage romances. In Boston there was a passing one with a nice woman from an old Boston family. I was invited to their home in Brookline a few times and to their Beacon Hill townhouse. A visit there at Christmas time was joyous, festive, and colorful; lots of people, punch bowls, candles, silver, and singing. But, although she and her family were very kind, the embryonic romance went nowhere.

There was a young woman whom I met through a college roommate. I spent a few weekends at her family's farm in their 1702 farmhouse. It was all original and crammed with antiques and old books. My girlfriend's mother, Mrs. Greenwood, had a large collection of early New England primers. I spent two Thanksgivings there. Once, instead of a turkey, the main dish was a large codfish with an apple in its mouth. The bowls were wooden, the plates and utensils pewter.

One cold winter day when the ruts in the muddy lane in front of the Greenwood house were frozen, I could not maneuver the big narrow front wheel of an 1890 bicycle I was riding. Over I went and broke my right arm. Dr. Greenwood was Chief of Dermatology at the Massachusetts General Hospital and had a private office on Marlborough Street, where he later instructed me in the practice of dermatology. He was a mild-mannered person who did not take himself or his profession too seriously. He told me that dermatology was a great specialty because once a patient, always a patient. All one needed to get started was a magnifying glass, a prescription pad, a bottle of lotion, and a jar of ointment. But, he said, be sure to have the patient bring back the jars or bottles at each appointment. Otherwise, at year's end, the patient would see the accumulated containers in the medicine closet and the rash unchanged.

During medical school, Betty French invited me out to the big Wellesley annual spring weekend called Barn Swallows because the festivities centered around a play their theater group produced. I do not recall how Betty and I met, but our relationship terminated at the entrance of her dormitory at the close of festivities. When I tried to kiss her goodbye she turned her cheek. It was distressing at the time but the best thing that could have happened. She may have had some interest in me, but turning the other cheek that fateful evening seemed to send me a message of disinterest. Years later I married Betty's classmate, Miriam "Monny" Barwood, and Betty sent us a pair of large silver serving spoons and a recording of Shubert's *Unfinished Symphony*, which we still have.

My deepest involvement was with a psychiatric social worker living at the Boston Psychopathic Hospital while I was working there. I do not recall whether I was "in love" or not, but I was right next to it until I danced with Miriam Barwood at a White Church square dance in Hanover in October of 1938. That encounter was it for me. So I hitchhiked both ways in the cold to and from Boston at Thanksgiving and broke off the relationship with the social worker. It was painful because she was a wonderful woman. This was the only romance that I broke up myself. The others just withered or the lady left me.

3

Harvard Medical School – 1934 to 1938

As my four years at Dartmouth came to a close I made the difficult decision to become a doctor. My decision was difficult because I could not separate my own wishes from those of my close friends who were all going to medical school. I was undoubtedly influenced by Dr. Harry French, who cared for me when I was near death with pneumonia.

I applied to medical school at the last minute in February of 1934 and was accepted to enter Harvard Medical School that fall on the condition that I take a stiff summer school course in biology and earn a grade of at least a B. That I did, in a long hot summer in New York City at Columbia University. I honestly don't know why I was admitted to Harvard. Maybe the initial interview with Dr. Worth Hale, the one-man admission committee, made the difference. I hobbled into his office for my interview with a long leg cast and crutches as a result of a serious ankle sprain I had suffered in the Carnival Snowshoe race. Six of us were accepted from Dartmouth and all except me made Alpha Omega Alpha, the distinction of being in the highest 10% of the graduating class.

I remained good friends in medical school with three of my Dartmouth buddies: Alfred Yankauer, Bub McAllister and Emerson Day. We were united by a common enemy: the pickled cadaver we dissected together. Yank never seemed to do much dissecting, but he always knew the answers when our anatomy professor, Dr. Robert Green, with flowing mustache and Shakespearean English, came around. After graduation McAllister went on to become the best vascular surgeon at Columbia Presbyterian Hospital in New York City. He was a smooth operator with the scalpel and with women. In spite of his living in the basement of a building in Copley Square, where he regularly shoveled coal, he always had a gorgeous creature on his arm. Yankauer worked in public health in New York state and for the United Nations, and became the long time editor of the American Journal of Public Health. Day performed some of the fundamental observations at Sloan-Kettering leading to the adoption of seat belts.

During my first year in medical school I was required to live in the new and lush Vanderbilt dormitory. These new digs stood in sharp contrast to Paul Magnuson's manure truck, parked at the curb, which my friends had used to move me in. My brilliant college friend, Emerson Day, was my roommate, and our relationship continued into later years. He also married a woman from Hanover, Ruth Fairfield, whose father was manager of the Hanover Inn.

I did well in medical school. Suddenly I was on a roll. I caught fire and got everything out of the Harvard Medical School that was possible for me to absorb. I went to school all year round except for one month in the summer when I was home with my parents. We had wonderful teachers. Imagine having John Enders, who subsequently received the Nobel Prize for growing the polio virus, and Hans Zinsser, the author of *Rats, Lice and History*, and *As I Remember Him*, looking down my old borrowed brass monocular microscope, helping me distinguish blue dots from red dots and trying to tell me what they meant; or Nobel Prize winner George Minot, sitting down in an old grungy Boston City Hospital ward with me and one other student as his only listeners while he took a dietary history from a man who lived on Washington Street, under the elevated railway tracks.

While in medical school I was totally absorbed in learning to be a doctor. I was either too busy or too tired to take much interest in extracurricular activities. I used the squash courts sometimes, and I rowed a few times on the Charles River in a single scull, imagining myself a budding Max Schmitt, as painted by Thomas Eakins, gliding alone on that beautiful and tranquil river on a crisp spring or fall day. On occasion I spent twenty-five cents to sit in the second balcony of Boston's Symphony Hall on a Saturday night. I didn't learn much about music but I enjoyed listening. Years later classical music "took", when I heard Benny Goodman play Mozart's Quintet in A. I figured there must be something to it, if Benny played it. On a Sunday morning a classmate, Charlie Hayden, might join me to listen to Reinhold Niebuhr, the distinguished Protestant scholar, and others of that ilk.

I had a job in the Vanderbilt Hall dining room. It was spacious and wood-paneled with high ceilings, brass chandeliers, and many windows. The flagstone floor felt hard by the end of the two-hour shifts, which I worked three times a day, Monday, Wednesday, and Friday. There were six of us waiters posted around the room, where we stood at attention in our crisp white jackets. Mrs. Robinson was the buxom, elderly woman in charge. There were no monkeyshines except one. Certain students always came in just as the dining room was closing; others were just SOB's who wore their college Phi Beta Kappa keys on their vests. For these obnoxious folks, we perfected the so-called napkin-to-ceiling maneuver: we placed a pat of butter in a folded napkin and then snapped it up to a spot on the ceiling above the intended target. The butter had to have enough consistency to hold it together but soft enough to stick to the ceiling. There it would slowly melt onto the victim's head.

One persistent latecomer was Dan Mooney. He was usually late for breakfast when we were anxious to get on with our day. At 8:25 am he routinely ordered two soft-boiled eggs, knowing that we waiters were required to cook and peel them to order. He became my nemesis; unfortunately he occasionally found bits of shells in his boiled eggs. When I came to practice in Fall River fourteen years later, there was Dan Mooney. He was now Chief of Surgery at St. Anne's Hospital and Union Hospital, the arch rival of my home base, Truesdale Hospital. After Mooney retired and left town, one of the doctors from St. Anne's told me that Mooney had regularly blocked my appointment at St. Anne's. Had it all begun years before with boiled eggshells?

During the three years I lived at the Boston Psychopathic Hospital, a teaching unit of HMS, I did laboratory work in exchange for room, board and laundry. Staying in school all year except for one month was not a chore. I took elective courses and did not feel put upon. I was having the time of my life. At the Psychopathic I could not go out of town. That was confining, but I learned a lot about central nervous system syphilis, tabes, and other mental diseases, most of which were beyond me. It gave me a good view of psychiatry and neurology of the time.

C. McPhee Campbell, a leader in his field, headed the hospital. We put patients in a tub, held them in with a canvas cover and ran hot or cold water through the tub. Occasionally we used large, almost hydrant-sized hoses. Some of the patients were confined singly in a locked room, stark naked with nothing but a rubber covered mattress. I had to go in to them to take their blood counts. I was nervous in the beginning but became used to it. For those poor folks who had gonorrhea or central nervous system syphilis, high temperature was the treatment at this Harvard teaching hospital. The patient was enclosed, except for his head, in a box and then the box temperature was cranked up to 104 or 105 degrees Fahrenheit. In Europe, Wagner Jauregg got a Nobel Prize for it. My recollection of this cruel and useless practice has always colored my view of medical care, much of which seems to be made up of fads. Remember Argerol, Mercurochrome, cupping, bloodletting? Even I was given sulfur and molasses, spring and fall, to thin or thicken my blood. Maybe that's why I like surgery. If one has a broken bone or a torn intestine or a ruptured ectopic pregnancy, the treatment has remained the same.

Although I was working at the Psychopathic and going to school, finances still fell short. I was forced to spend precious time earning money instead of taking advantage of the tremendous learning experiences available to a Harvard medical student. But I couldn't complain. I had a place to eat and sleep, a medical library, and the world famous Peter Bent Brigham Hospital all within two blocks. Some of my classmates had to leave school to keep the home fires burning.

I added to my workload by taking a job investigating the credit worthiness of clients applying for any kind of insurance. Each morning I drove to the office of the Retail Credit Company in an old 1930 Model A Ford. I don't remember how I happened to have the use of it. I picked up slips with clients' data and toured my territory in and around Waltham and Brookline. I was surprised and distressed to see how easily neighbors talked about the intimate lives of their friends. The next morning I turned in my reports and collected new slips.

One person I could not locate had given his address as the corner of two busy streets in Brighton. There I found a large saloon with a huge mirror on the wall against which all the liquor was displayed. In front ran the usual long polished wooden bar. To my inquires all I got was blank stares, more vigorous polishing of glasses and statements of "never heard of him." Six weeks later he was found dead in a gravel pit. Too bad his widow never received the $75,000 policy he had applied for.

Some time in my third year at Harvard, I had come to the end of my finances. Loans, jobs, and everything else had not yielded enough. I was disconsolate. Then, unexpectedly, my brother Bill showed up at the outpatient department of the Peter Bent Brigham Hospital for a visit. If it hadn't been for him, I would never have finished Harvard Medical School. He had just received a good-sized bonus check from his World War I service, something like $400 or $500. He endorsed the check to me, took a trolley outside in Brigham Circle and disappeared. I didn't see him again for probably five years.

Bill and I were close emotionally, but our actual contact was minimal. I never forgot his generosity to me at a time when he himself was broke. Happily, I was able to repay this concrete expression of friendship a few times later and was with him constantly for the last two weeks of his life when he was dying from pancreatic cancer in a Veterans Hospital in New Jersey.

The year 1936 was the three hundredth anniversary of Harvard University celebrated in Harvard Yard in Cambridge. It was the gala of all galas. I was an usher because they paid us medical students two dollars. The academic procession began with a representative of the oldest university, in Egypt, I think, followed by the others in chronological order in their splendid and colorful robes and accoutrements. It was impressive. I was standing near the entrance to the V.I.P. seats when President Franklin Roosevelt's car pulled up. It was a black sedan and I think he was in the front seat. I was standing fifteen or twenty feet from him as he turned his torso, lower legs dangling out of the car. An aid straightened his legs as FDR shot the metal braces down and he was helped to his feet. He put on his top hat and walked easily to his seat in the heavy mist with a man by his side, not obviously holding him. Although I was in street clothes and wore no official identification, I experienced no interference from the few secret service men in evidence. There must have been many around, but Roosevelt appeared to be treated like any other attendee.

While at Harvard, I was fortunate to be able to do my surgical clerkship at Boston's Peter Bent Brigham Hospital, now called Brigham and Women's Hospital. The Brigham had been built in 1912 in the pavilion style to avoid the transmission of infection. It consisted of five two-story buildings connected by an open Pike on one end, and had a tennis court in the space between each building. When I arrived in 1934, the Brigham was full of stories of the noted brain surgeon, Harvey Cushing, who had just been forcibly retired because of age, a rule that he himself had instituted years earlier. The word was that when he came down the Pike, students and house staff scattered because he took them on to the wards and grilled them on any patient he chose.

During my surgical clerkship at the Brigham, Dr. David Cheever, a genteel Boston Brahmin, was one of my role models. Even now I recall with gratitude how gently he performed one of those huge mastectomy dressings on a patient in the Peter Bent Brigham amphitheater in front of a first-year class of 150 students. Emerson Day, my roommate and still a good friend, turned green but didn't hit the floor. It seems that from then on, I wanted to be like Dr. Cheever. As a fourth-year student, I was a substitute intern at the Brigham and was Dr. Cheever's first assistant on a cholecystectomy, the first operation he did when he returned from an enforced year in Arizona because of arthritis. Frank Lepreau, a fourth year student, first assisting Dr. David Cheever--that was my Matterhorn.

Although Dr. Cheever and his first dressing may have been the seed, my surgical aspirations grew because of the surgical house staff at the Brigham: Bert Dunphy, Robert Gross, Stanley Hoerr, Richard Warren, Bart Quigley, Carl Walters. They all went on to distinguished careers in academic surgery. Gross, in 1938, as an assistant resident did the first successful ligation of the ductus arteriosus, when the chief, Dr. William Ladd, was out of town thus inaugurating the era of surgical repair of congenital defects of the heart and great vessels. Can you imagine Robert Gross in his immaculate whites from top to toe checking my own histories and physicals? That was a trip even before he became so famous.

There was surgery at the Peter Bent Brigham and medicine at the Boston City Hospital, where the Thorndike laboratory men were making names for themselves: Wesley Spink, the great William Castle, Thomas Hale Ham, Soma Weiss, Henry Jackson, Chester Keefer, Max Finland, and the Nobelist, Dr. George Minot. Lewis Thomas was one or two years ahead of me and was already marked as a great. In his book, *The Youngest Science*, he wrote about his Boston City Hospital experience and the patients we all saw in the days before antibiotics.

The role model influence was strong and surgery became my ultimate career, affording me great satisfaction. Surgery requires a combination of intellectual judgment, technical skill, basic scientific knowledge, and compassion all centered on a suffering human being whose recovery was the only compensation. How satisfying it is to take someone hanging on the edge and bring her back whole; to have the parents look at you with a lovely smile and say, "Thank you, Doctor." Vanity, vanity, all is vanity, ego trip and all that, but there it is. Also one could *do something*, unlike the physician in Fildes' painting who could only sit by the child's bedside and worry. As a surgeon I could remove an appendix and in a week the patient would be jumping rope again, unless she had rheumatic fever or another dire medical disease.

In addition to my mentors, many other influences played a role in my philosophy of medical practice. There was the two-volume biography of Doctor William Osler by Doctor Harvey Cushing; the volume on Harvey Cushing by Doctor John Fulton; Osler's *Alabama Student and Other Biographical Essays, Aequanimitas,* and then a small volume called *Doctor and Patient* by Francis W. Peabody, a famous 1907 graduate of Harvard Medical School. Dr. Peabody wrote his essays while at that germinating center of young physicians, the Thorndike Memorial Laboratory at the Boston City Hospital. It isn't just his well-known essay entitled "The Care of the Patient." There are several others that are moving, plus a remarkable introduction by the great Hans Zinsser.

One of Peabody's essays, called "The Soul of the Clinic," is a letter in response to a request by Warfield Longcope who was then at Hopkins asking for advice on how to run a medical clinic. The subject turns on whether one should have a part-time or full-time faculty. Peabody replies with something like, "It is the manner of men you pick, not the system and law that kills but more of the spirit that gives life." He died of stomach cancer in 1927 at the age of 46.

Beginning a new life

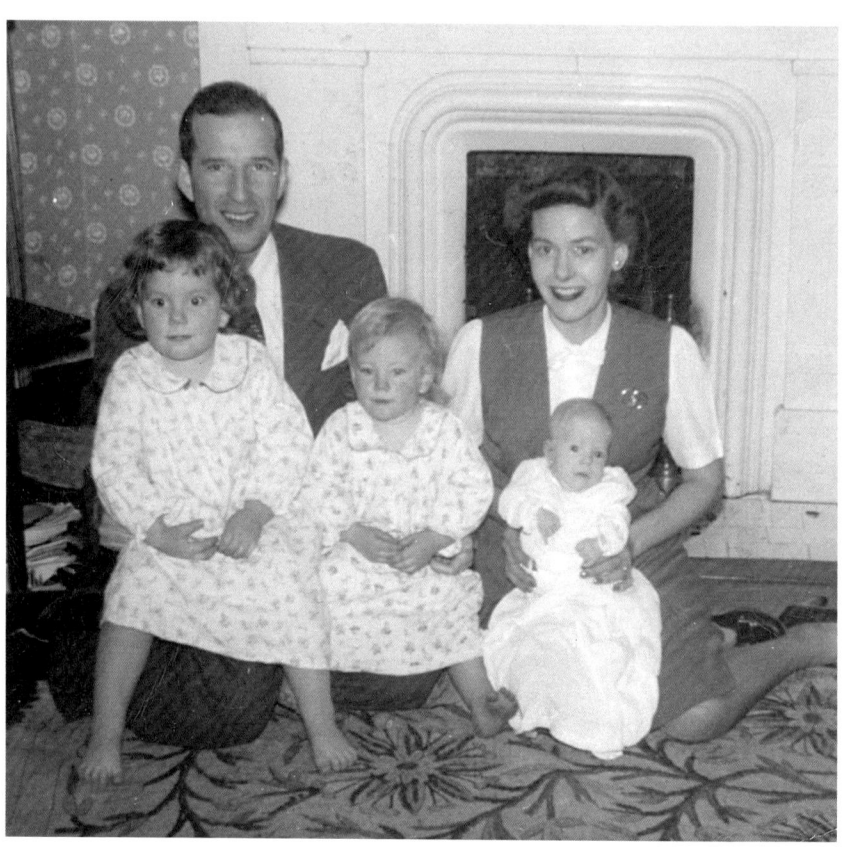

Three Under 3
Lucy Ann, Judy and Sue
Christmas 1944

4

Hanover and Yale

I thought a disaster had occurred when I did not get a surgical internship at the Peter Bent Brigham Hospital. In those days throughout the country the choice internship appointments were made in the fall on no prescribed date. The good Boston appointments were made in January at the latest. So, as in my case, if one failed to get a Boston job, he was hung out to dry. I figured that I might end up in some foreign place like Fall River or New Bedford, Massachusetts, in both of which I eventually practiced.

I looked in the Dartmouth Alumni Register and found the name of Dr. Howard Clute, a prominent Boston surgeon and Chairman at Boston University. Lamenting my fate, I stopped at his office to tell him my story. He picked up the phone and called Dr. Jay Gile, a trustee of Dartmouth, an old medical school classmate, and good personal friend, saying, "I've a young man here with his tail between his legs thinking the end of the world has come. Can you do anything for him?"

Within a week I had a nonpaying position in the pathology department of the Dartmouth Medical School, a room in the attic of Professor Ralph Miller's house, meals at the hospital, and his bicycle to get there. Again I had a great time. I was performing autopsies all over the state, in featherbeds in farmhouse bedrooms, back rooms in the local funeral home or any unoccupied place available. Indeed, I graduated from the ivory tower of the Harvard Medical School one Saturday at noon and at 9:00 the next morning, I was touring the streets of Woodsville, New Hampshire, with a slightly more experienced colleague and my carpenter's box of autopsy tools in hand. We found the local furniture store on the main street, pulled down the green shades in the showroom, pushed back the furniture, rolled up the rug, laid down a lot of newspapers, and did the autopsy.

I once searched out a patient's son in order to get permission for an autopsy on his father who had died at the Mary Hitchcock Hospital. I found him chopping wood in a lot high on a mountain, 75 miles from Hanover. In those days a high autopsy rate was a marker for the quality of care in a hospital and figured prominently in the overall evaluation of an institution. Mary Hitchcock Hospital, at 85 percent, had one of the highest rates in the country. Sadly, because of the time and expense the pathologist requires, autopsies are rare nowadays.

The major dividend of losing my Boston appointment was coming to Hanover where I met my wife, Miriam Barwood. As is so often said, but I say it here with many underlines, "It was the best thing that ever happened to me." Fifty-two years later after a celebration *a deux* in our home on New Year's Eve, 1991, I could have said the same.

Monny and I were married on October 8, 1939 at the White Church in Hanover, New Hampshire. In attendance were our parents, all of Monny's siblings, several of her local and Wellesley friends and a few college and medical school friends of mine. I was apprehensive about what pranks my friends might have planned for us newlyweds, so I insisted that Monny and I leave after spending only a short time at the reception in the church hall where we had first danced. This was my first mistake in our married life. Appropriately Monny had wished to stay, dance and socialize with our guests.

Further marring the first days of our marriage, just two days after our wedding, I had an appointment with Dr. Samuel C. Harvey, the professor and chairman of the Department of Surgery at Yale regarding my application for an appointment as a surgical intern. In those days interns and residents had no choice about vacation. In Hanover, I was told when I could take mine and had arranged my marriage and interview dates around the allotted vacation.

Unfortunately Dr. Harvey was attending the funeral of Dr. Harvey Cushing, the world's greatest neurosurgeon and I was told to await the second-in-command, Dr. Gustaf Lindskog. I waited and waited and waited. Finally after several hours I emerged to join Monny, who had also waited. She sat in the car, wearing her new wool suit in the boiling sun of Cedar Street — not exactly an auspicious introduction to married life but perhaps a taste of what to expect when one marries a physician. Our belated honeymoon at the "Shack" in Brewster on Cape Cod Bay was delicious and carefree. These years, 1938 to 1940, were happy ones for me — a year in rural pathology followed by 12 months of a rotating internship capped by my wooing and winning Miriam Barwood all took place in the town so beloved by its Dartmouth alumni.

Shortly after we were married, my wife's father, Arthur Barwood, came down at our invitation for a Sunday morning breakfast. He found me cutting out figures from the comics. What kind of a man married my daughter, he must have thought. He was mollified when he learned I was trying to improve my surgical technique by using my left hand.

In Hanover we had two rooms at 10 Pleasant Street near my wife's parents, who had occupied the same two rooms when they were first married. Our tiny stove and washbowl made up the kitchen. After the first roast fused to the pan, Monny soon prepared her usual elegant small meal for two with candles, wedding-present china and silver.

This two-story wooden building where we first lived was the same structure where, in 1796, Nathan Smith, the founder of the Dartmouth Medical School, delivered his first lectures. Smith later founded the Yale School of Medicine where I was Assistant Clinical Professor of Surgery. Continuing my connection with Smith, in 1996, the New England Surgical Society awarded me their occasional Nathan Smith Award for Surgical Excellence. A previous recipient was Joseph Murray who performed the first successful kidney transplant at the Peter Bent Brigham Hospital in Boston in 1964 for which he received the Nobel Prize. Obviously I am not in the Murray stratosphere, but I was pleased to be recognized as a good clinical surgeon and teacher.

Monny continued to be a lab technician, going north to Littleton or south to Claremont, as well as at the Hitchcock Clinic in Hanover. We were often separated because she was intermittently sent to those places, but we needed her income as I was paid a negligible sum.

Thanks to Dawson Tyson, a consummate surgeon at the Mary Hitchcock, I obtained a surgical internship at Yale, one of the best programs in the country. This was an internship, meaning that I was at the bottom of the training ladder for two more years. But that was a price I was glad to pay for this prestigious appointment. The program was based on the old Hopkins and Brigham pyramidal system where eight interns started out, and after four years, if one was lucky or good enough, that one became the resident surgeon for a year, responsible for the whole ward service and, in a distant but still tangible way, for the care of private patients too. One was truly king of the hill and could operate on any ward patient at any time of the day. If you made it to the top, Samuel C. Harvey, a brilliant but remote figure, suddenly came to know you. He was always accessible, sympathetic, and he freely shared his encyclopedic knowledge.

So off we went to New Haven, and the move proved to be a jolt to both Monny and me. We borrowed an open truck from Monny's high school friends and took our furniture to New Haven in two trips. We looked like Okies. Everything was tied on with ropes. I had the steering wheel to hold on to, but Monny had nothing. So this Wellesley bride bounced around in the springless cab like popcorn in the making. What a woman! She now had to become a city girl and was so pleased when we found a first-floor railroad apartment abutting an empty lot full of weeds. I was not there much because I was "on" every other night and weekend, which meant being in the hospital and sleeping there. And, no matter what the schedule showed, one was never actually off until one's work was done.

Monny secured a job as an all-purpose technician, secretary, chaperone and receptionist with Dr. Chunky Robbins, an undistinguished general practitioner who nonetheless had a carriage trade practice. One of his affluent patients was Mrs. Ogden Miller, the wife of a Yale recruiter. Anne Miller, in March 1942, became the first patient in the United States to be treated successfully with penicillin. She had had a spontaneous infected miscarriage and was in extremis when she was saved by the miracle mold. Hers was the classic demonstration of the old boy network. Dr. John Fulton, Professor of Physiology at the Yale Medical School was an ardent Yalie and a Rhodes scholar with Howard Florey. Florey and Boris Chain were the joint discoverers of the antibacterial properties of penicillin. The tiny amount of penicillin in the United States was in the care of Dr. Chester Keefer, a Harvard Medical School professor. Dr. Francis Blake, a Harvard Medical School alumnus and infectious disease specialist, was Mrs. Miller's hospital physician. These Harvard and Yale alumni succeeded in getting enough minuscule doses of penicillin to save their patient. Mrs. Miller lived to be 90 years old, dying in 1999.

All of us on the resident staff were excited and the interns and residents were often up all night to give the quite painful injections of the crystalline substance. One of them, Bob Johnston, somewhat bleary-eyed from lack of sleep, had to present Mrs. Miller's case to a full amphitheater including the discoverer of penicillin, Alexander Fleming, in the front row. It soon became known that much penicillin passed into the urine unaltered. Because of the short supply of penicillin, we house officers collected the urine in bedpans and urinals, poured it into bottles and sent it off to the chemical companies in northern New Jersey so the excess penicillin could be recovered and returned as a lifesaving golden powder. As part of a search for the best penicillin mold, the United States Air Force was directed to bring back samples of earth from wherever they went. The best variety was found on a moldy cantaloupe in Peoria, Illinois.

The discovery of antibiotics by Alexander Fleming in 1928, published in 1929, and the demonstration of the therapeutic properties of penicillin by Florey and Chain in the early 1940's, must join W. T. G. Morton's introduction of ether anesthesia in 1846 and Louis Pasteur's germ theory of disease in the 1860's as being among the greatest contributions to human health up to now. Penicillin came just in time to save thousands of Allied soldiers in World War II. Just think: before that magic powder was available, a tiny cut on the playground or a laceration opening a can in the kitchen could have spelled death.

As a Yale intern I covered the Emergency Room and the ambulance. One of the first calls I answered came at night from the New Haven Railroad Station. A trainman had had both legs severed above the knee by a rolling car. I found him in the cab of a steam engine where his associates had used the bell cord from the locomotive as a life saving tourniquet on his upper thighs. The runaway car had come off the "hump," an elevated area in the yards where unmanned cars were rolled down to link up with other cars when a train was being made up.

Also about this time, to the delight of my colleagues, I spent one night in jail. My friends came down to the local New Haven police station and laughed at me through the bars. It was a case of mistaken identity and I was freed in the morning but I was definitely on the police blotter.

At this time the house staff was busy learning and performing surgery and we loved it. Occasionally Samuel C. Harvey, after his nap in the afternoon, would go out to the hospital courts and play tennis. Another of my idols was L. C. Foster, known as Stem. He was a beautiful technical surgeon without fuss. All of a sudden the operation would be over. If the case finished around noon he'd say, "Let's go have some lunch." We'd get into his long Brewster green automobile, and have lunch at Mory's. I felt like the crown prince.

As Montaigne says, "One learns much good and bad just from observing others with whom one has little or no contact." This was so with Larry Crowley. He was an ordinary third or fourth-year Yale medical student when I was going through the residency. He did his work, but I do not recall him as a brilliant or unusually dexterous surgeon. He married a beautiful woman who was a Yale nurse and Crowley became a Yale-New Haven surgical intern. Then disaster struck. His young wife contracted severe paralytic poliomyelitis. From beneath his ordinariness, his true character shone brightly. Crowley dropped his opportunity for advancement to chief surgical resident at Yale and the promise of an academic career, to follow his wife to Warm Springs, Georgia, for a prolonged period. He arranged his life to care for her while carrying on a much less glamorous surgical career in the Veterans Administration Hospitals. Virtue had its reward. His wife remained somewhat crippled, but she could get around and made a contribution to nursing when they eventually settled in Palo Alto. In California Lawrence

Crowley became one of the better deans of the Stanford University Medical School, which he helped raise to national prominence.

~

When Monny was six months pregnant with Lucy Ann, I took her to see my childhood home in Hastings and to New York City. She was game but it was hard on her starting with the wild ride on the roller coaster at Rye Beach. With my German buddies next door we went to a ball game at the Polo Grounds, at that time the home stadium of the New York Giants. The game starred Frankie Frisch, the Fordham flash at 2nd base whose name was on my baseball bat. It was a hot day for my young wife who knew and cared nothing about baseball and who had to listen to the rowdy crowd and the constant yells of "Hey! I've got hot dogs!" Finally we danced on the Astor Roof to Harry James, which was a distinct pleasure for her. For better or worse, she had learned something about her husband's background.

After a year in the apartment on Park Street in New Haven, we moved into free hospital accommodations—two rooms on the second floor of an old brick row house on a busy corner across the street from the hospital. We had quite a time adjusting to the noise of the traffic when we were trying to sleep. It was also hot. There were four families in the three-story building. We all shared one kitchen and two of us shared one bathroom. The ladies were tolerant and there were no crises. The living became tight for Monny, however, when she soon had two, then three children in two rooms, and she was still working. It was around this time that Judy fell down stairs. We had her head x-rayed and were surprised to see innumerable cracks in her skull from previous falls. Judy has since grown to be a fine woman, in spite of, or perhaps because of, these numerous bumps to the head.

We hired a baby-sitter while Monny was bringing in the cash. I made nothing for two years and $40 a month for two more years. Then for one year as the all-powerful resident surgeon at the Yale-New Haven Hospital, my salary rose to one hundred dollars a month. Uniforms, meals, and hospital housing were provided. I had no complaint because I was learning all the time and absorbed in mastering the surgical craft. For my wife, though, it must have been a chore coping with the care of three children, continuing to work and missing an often-absent husband. She never complained.

Being completely broke, I asked for a loan from two affluent private surgeons in New Haven for whom I worked, but no dice. Next I asked Johnny Mendillo whose practice served those who lived across the tracks and were mostly Italian. His immediate response was, "Sure, Frank! How much?" I asked for $5,000 to start and maybe $5,000 later. The interview took place under a street light on the sidewalk across from the hospital. A check came the next day. I immediately took out my first insurance policy for $10,000 with Dr. John Mendillo the beneficiary.

Memories from this time in New Haven are many. At Christmas in 1941, I trudged home in the snow carrying our first big Christmas present, a record player in a nice wooden case. It had cost me $25 dollars. One Sunday morning in the spring, Monny and I, carrying

Lucy Ann in a basket, took a trolley car out to the vicinity of Sleeping Giant State Park for a picnic. The basket and Lucy became a burden so we left her on the side of the path for the hour it took us to complete our hike up the hill and return.

In New Haven, my wife and I and three children were interviewed by Dr. Lorrin A. Shepard for a job in the Middle East. Dr. Shepard was highly esteemed in medical missionary circles. He offered me a job as his associate successor at the American Hospital in Istanbul. This was a flattering and attractive offer, as I had been thinking about missionary work for a long time. I might have accepted if we hadn't had three young children. At that time there were several people on the house staff at New Haven, fine men and women who had been brought up as missionary children. Air transport wasn't common in those days so the families would be in China or Africa for five years at a clip without returning to the United States. These children, now my contemporaries, seemed mixed up. They didn't know if they were Chinese or American or Congolese. We didn't want to take that risk with our own children, so we turned the offer down.

I had just been appointed resident surgeon in the spring of 1944 when I was offered a job as general and thoracic surgeon at the Hitchcock Clinic in Hanover, New Hampshire, with a continued deferment. It was hard to refuse because I loved Hanover so much; but I did, and wisely so. In the early spring of 1945 I had my physical and was in New York City with my papers, ready to get my military uniform when the war ended.

I never did service in the military, although I was designated plastic surgeon for the crippled children's program for the state of Connecticut because most of the regular physicians were off in the war. I think this appointment happened as a result of my work in the aftermath of the Hartford Circus fire, which occurred on July 6, 1944. Many died and hundreds were severely burned. Because Hartford had a small house staff, some of my colleagues and I, who had quite a bit of experience with burns and skin grafting, went up there for a month of intense doctoring on these burn patients.

Following my residency, I stayed on as a junior faculty member at $2,500 a year. We lived in a nice rented house in Fairhaven on the east side of New Haven. I commuted by trolley car after trying bicycling to save money. Grand Avenue was too busy and I was not about to be crushed between cars. We ate a lot of mackerel at nineteen cents a pound. This was a decision year for us, mostly for me. Coming home from the long white-coat life of conferences, clinical presentations, and occasional luncheons with international notables and department chairmen only to find my lovely Monny down in the cellar, hand-wringing out sheets in the set tubs was intolerable. To make it in academic medicine one had to do research and publish, neither one of which was my forte. I am a teacher and patient care type. So my move into a private practice career with some teaching turned out to be a wise decision.

I often returned to New Haven for events and to visit old colleagues and usually brought a striped bass in ice for my host. On February 17, 1951 I gathered twelve of Dr. Harvey's ex-resident surgeons at the New Haven Lawn Club in honor of his retirement and to unveil his portrait by his good friend, Deane Keller. It was a jovial evening with men from far away in the United States and

Canada. From Westport I brought white carnations for everyone. We established a small "encouragement" fund for an assistant resident to stay in the program. In 1961 the grant was $150.

We also provided the seed money for an annual Samuel C. Harvey Lectureship on the history of surgery. This brought distinguished men to New Haven for a pleasant evening, beginning with the lecture in the Yale Medical Historical Library and then adjourning to a small dinner at Mory's with entertainment by the Whiffenpoofs. I gave one lecture, as did Dr. William L. Glenn, who had kept the project alive for 25 years. At that 25th year about 20 of us came to dinner and found at our places a small white oblong box tied with a blue ribbon. Inside mine I found a coin silver spoon with the maker's name, N. Harding, clearly shown. Also in lighter engraving was "F. J. L. Jr. 3-3-80". Bill, in his usual well-chosen words, said, "I have collected these spoons over the years, but now it is my privilege to give them to my most appropriate friends, fellow surgeons who work with their hands as did the artisans who made each spoon." It was an emotional moment.

Each lecturer was given a book from Doctor Harvey's library. I received *Surgical Observations on Tumours with Cases and Operations* by John Collins Warren, Professor of Anatomy and Surgery at Harvard University and Surgeon of the Massachusetts General Hospital, Boston 1837. Dr. Warren was the surgeon who, on October 16, 1846, performed the operation at the first public demonstration of anesthesia in the still existing amphitheater at the Massachusetts General Hospital. As I write this, I have that book in hand with the date of my lecture on tuberculosis — March 9, 1970. On that date, as I entered the library at 4 p.m. to prepare my exhibits, I was amazed to find my youngest daughter, Mimi, then 16 years old, up from Westtown School for my lecture.

5

Getting Started

The months before I started practice in New Bedford were a mixture of pleasure and angst. Monny and I spent that summer in the town of Brewster on Cape Cod Bay with its long flats extending out into the bay a half-mile or more. It was an idyllic setting, but I could not suppress my anxiety about our situation. I had no license to practice in Massachusetts, and so I was not working. I had to wait until September or October when the Massachusetts Board of Registration met to officially approve my license with reciprocity from the state of Connecticut. Money was short. I cut my fingers digging on the flats for razor clams, which often provided us with food during those otherwise lovely summer months.

My college friend, Dr. Paul Magnuson, had told me there was a need for a thoracic surgeon in New Bedford and so we moved there. With the encouragement of Dr. Curtis Tripp, a Dartmouth alumnus and chief of surgery in the hospital, I slowly got started. My first patient was a prominent man about town who was a lawyer and later became a judge. I drained an abscess on his buttock, which had followed an injection of penicillin. He became a good friend and promoter. In surgical practice those days, one had to take out "lumps and bumps," drain abscesses and sew up lacerations at 3:00 a.m. in the emergency room and hope that someday you would get a real case like a patient with appendicitis or one with gallstones.

We rented a house on Hawthorne Street in New Bedford, and I had my office upstairs above our apartment. Later I had real office space on the busiest corner in New Bedford at Union and Pleasant Streets. It was on the second floor above a popular drug store run by Cliff Higham. I thought the location in the center of town and above the drugstore would attract patients. I still have the wooden shingle that was nailed to the door on the street leading to the upstairs office. It says "F. J. Lepreau M.D. Waiting Room." The announcement in the paper read, "Frank J. Lepreau, M.D. announces the opening of his office for the practice of general and thoracic surgery at 528 Pleasant Street. Dial 2-2952." That was the extent of the publicity I ran once in the *New Bedford Standard Times* announcing my entrance to practice in New Bedford. There was no financial subsidy around then, and there was no group supportive financial arrangement. I was on my own, in solo, independent practice like most other beginning practitioners of the time.

While I set up my office, Monny made curtains and johnnies and sewed up sheets for the examining table while continuing her work as a technician and running the household. Since she was making money as a laboratory technician, she employed Tillie, a happy, young Polish girl who took care of the three girls. They liked her and she liked them. We bought two used tricycles for Lucy Ann, aged 5, and Judy, aged 4 and a simpler set of wheels in pale green for Suzy who was 3. While we were living at Hawthorne Street, Lucy Ann came down with scarlet fever. The Public Health

Department posted a large red sign on our house proclaiming the presence of scarlet fever within.

There wasn't much activity in the office. I spent a lot of time reading the paper. The adjoining office holder was a nose and throat physician who had had an alcohol problem but was in recovery. He was kind. Occasionally he would bring a mother and child by the hand and say, "There is a new doctor in town who is a specialist in heart and lung conditions. I want him to check your child's heart and lungs to make sure he is suitable for anesthesia when I take out his tonsils." He would seat the couple in my empty office and I'd do a heart and lung exam and maybe take a blood pressure and get $5. Perhaps that is the origin of my affection for alcoholics.

I presume that because of our friendship with Dr. and Mrs. Paul Magnuson, who had high professional and social standing in the community, we were welcomed into that same group. The nursing school on the grounds of St. Luke's Hospital held numerous dances and other social functions. At a waltz night contest held around the holidays, Monny and I won the prize as the best waltzers.

We became close friends of Dr. Carl Persons and his wife. Persons was a Harvard Medical School graduate of 1917 and a man of impeccable character. He had severe Marie-Strumpels disease, a total fusion of the spine. Indeed if he were lying flat on his back, he would be unable to turn over. Despite his affliction he was a great golfer and a wonderful person. He had a wide-ranging socioeconomic general practice. No matter who the doctor entering the community, whether he had graduated from Middlesex or Harvard, Dr. Persons would send one of his best patients to the new doctor to help him get started. He did that for me.

When the famed William Osler of Johns Hopkins described the ideal general practitioner he could have been describing Dr. Persons. Some of Osler's essays are incorporated in his *Aequanimitas*, published in 1904 when he was Regis Professor at Oxford. A similar collection of essays, *Doctor and Patient*, by Dr. Francis W. Peabody was published in 1930 and continues to be quoted. They contributed to my maturing as a physician. In recognition of all the qualities mentioned by Osler and Peabody, Perry Culver, H.M.S. 1941, and I had Peabody's book republished and given to several generations of Harvard Medical School students. Along the way I made a pleasant relationship with the big Bill Castle, H.M.S. 1921, and Peabody's widow, Mrs. George C. Shattuck.

In New Bedford, the hospital and medical staff were good to me. I was immediately put on the surgical ward service with Dr. Joseph Ponte as my chief. He was a quiet, authoritative figure, the surgeon for almost all the Portuguese patients in the city. One evening I was dressed up in a tuxedo at a nurses' dance on the grounds. Dr. Ponte appeared and politely asked me about a young adult on the service suspected of having appendicitis. Fortunately I could tell him that I had just left the bedside; I knew exactly what was going on and planned to check on him again in a very short time.

I did the first pulmonary resection ever done in that city. It was a lobectomy for bronchiectasis diagnosed with the now archaic technique of using lipiodol and local anesthesia. The patient had a good result.

St. Luke's, the main hospital in town, had no morbidity-mortality conference. I profited from my past experience as a pathologist by gaining employment at the hospital as assistant pathologist at $75 a month. I did some nice surgery and my cases did well. I was treated well professionally. In the hospital after I left, it was said that Dr. Tripp made me unwelcome, but that was not true.

~

    After seven or eight months I became disenchanted with solo practice, not necessarily because of New Bedford. I found that solo practice was too competitive. I preferred to work in a group practice where all shared the same amenities and problems. About this time I was invited by Dr. Warren Atwood, a Dartmouth and Harvard Medical school graduate, to join him and others in a loose group of congenial doctors at the Truesdale Clinic in Fall River. Thanks to these men and to the community, I enjoyed a fine practice in Fall River and Westport. I had several firsts in the area such as patent ductus, mitral valve procedures, sympathectomy, pulmonary resections, plastic procedures, cleft palate and lips. In the late 1940s and 50s, the assistant residents from Boston University rotated through our surgical service. I enjoyed working with them and teaching them. They did about 75 percent of my private cases, which was heresy back then, even if I was always present from skin to skin. We all had a good time and the patients had excellent post-operative care.
    Dr. Atwood was my hero. After medical school he had trained at several hospitals, among them the Women's Free Hospital in Brookline, which catered to the more affluent patients and where fourth-year Harvard Medical students, including me, learned to do outpatient gynecology and pelvic examinations. In fact

Women's Free Hospital was where I met Dr. John Rock, a Harvard Medical professor, who, in spite of his Catholicism, became the point man for the acceptance of the contraceptive pill.

When the invitation came to join Dr. Atwood at the Truesdale Clinic, I was delighted to move. He was a gentle, pleasant man who had succeeded as chairman of Department of Surgery after the death of Dr. Philemon Truesdale. The clinic had undergone a tumultuous period following the loss of Dr. Truesdale's strong leadership and authoritarian ways. Now with character, surgical skill, sound judgment and honesty, Dr. Atwood became the new leader of the group. He had done a tremendous amount of obstetrics during the war years when he was the only obstetrician around. I once watched him successfully deliver a baby from a woman coming off the street with a prolapsed cord. He did a version, turning the infant around and extracting it feet first, getting the baby out smoothly. It was a situation that required great manual skill, and Atwood was a consummate and smooth technician.

I inherited his non-obstetrical patients when he was off call or out of town. Although I never did transurethral prostatic resections, I was prepared for any urological condition because of my nine months in New Haven on the urology service under Clyde Deming, one of Hugh Young's star residents of Johns Hopkins. I assisted Dr. Atwood in surgery and carefully followed his cases. We had a good relationship. I am ever grateful to him and he is still one of my heroes. Later on he developed tuberculosis and had to spend almost a year at a sanatorium in the Adirondacks. Unfortunately his return was marred by stressful marital problems.

I found the Truesdale Hospital a relaxed and special place to work. The group of surgeons and nursing staff functioned as if they were a family. We started a journal club with all the appurtenances of a high-quality general surgical service with residents. My practice was taking off and I was having a great time.

Located in the Highlands area of the city, the hospital had solariums on the riverside providing an open and relaxing area for those patients who were well enough to sit there. The operating suite on the top floor had a expansive view of the Taunton River. There were three operating rooms. Dr. Atwood had the central room. Dr. Cornelius Hawes, a competent, Harvard-trained general surgeon, worked in Room #2, which was a little smaller. Dr. Daniel Gallery and I alternately shared the third room. Dr. Gallery was a gregarious, loveable Irishman who had thoracic surgery training in Montreal, spending time there with the renowned and notorious Dr. Norman Bethune, who was the subject of a lovely novel titled *The Watch That Ends the Night,* by Hugh MacLennan.

It is hard to imagine now that I, as a new young surgeon, could go to Truesdale Hospital on Tuesdays, Thursdays and Saturdays and begin my list at eight in the morning and stay all day until the cases were finished. Dr. Gallery did the same thing on Mondays, Wednesdays and Fridays, and of course Dr. Hawes and Dr. Warren Atwood were working daily beginning at 8 o'clock in the morning in their own operating rooms. Dr. Charlie Bryan, who had been one year ahead of me at Harvard, became a close friend. He was a brilliant, albeit gloomy person, and an outstanding radiologist.

The predecessor of the hospital was the Truesdale Clinic built in 1914 on Rock Street in the center of town. When I arrived in 1948 I was given upstairs rooms with a large consulting room complete with a working fireplace. In winter I brought in wood and frequently had a fire. Ray Hadfield crafted built-in closets and bookcases, and Monny, as always, made the curtains and more johnnies. Professionally it couldn't have been better.

At an appropriate time in the afternoon my wonderful secretary, Mrs. Alice Kret, served tea. She sat in a small corner behind a banister in the hall where she did all her work. Alice was a great asset to my practice and a striking example of how important it is for a physician to have someone intelligent and courteous as his right hand person in the office.

In 1958, Norman Cousins, editor of the *Saturday Review of Literature*, brought 27 Polish women who had been used as experimental animals by the Nazis to the United States for rehabilitation. In 1959 he brought eight more. Our Friends Meeting took Marya and Zosia, two of these Ravensbrueck lapins, as they were called. I took responsibility for their medical care. Only one required hospitalization–her tibia had been opened and potent toxic bacteria had been inserted. I cleaned it up and after several weeks closed the wound.

Why mention it here? Because it could not have happened without the very Polish Alice Kret. She and I and Casimir Babiarz of the *Fall River Herald News* drove to New York City to bring the women back to Fall River. Alice made all the housing and social arrangements. As is so often the case when one is involved even in a small way with these do-good projects, I met wonderful people. In New York City at supper in the Mayflower

Hotel we met several high profile philanthropists besides
Cousins. I recall Erica Anderson, a marvelous human
being and in the top tier of New York City
photographers. She was friend and official photographer
to Dr. Albert Schweitzer for fifteen years. As such, she
had come to the Mellons' hospital in Haiti, named after
Schweitzer, and she became friends with Monny and me.
We later had two pleasant overnight visits at her
retirement home in Great Barrington, Massachusetts,
which she called the Albert Schweitzer Friendship
House. Among many Schweitzer artifacts are 30,000
Schweitzer negatives stored in a climate-controlled area.
Before her death in 1976, Erica gave me several beautiful
8 x 10 photos of Hôpital Albert Schweitzer and an
autographed photograph of her and Dr. Schweitzer.

One holiday season, Alice and her husband,
Edward, invited me to join them on a project of the Fall
River Junior Chamber of Commerce. The JC's had
assembled a group of poor children and provided each
one with five dollars to be spent on Christmas gifts. We
took each child individually on a shopping spree, and
most bought presents for their mothers. We then
gathered together after the shopping and the wives of the
men helped the children wrap their purchases.

Edward Kret died of a myocardial infarction at
age 35 leaving Alice with two small children. Alice
remained my ever-present professional and personal
associate, much beloved by our children and extremely
kind to my mother while I was in Haiti. My patients
loved her. She knew them all by name; she was always
pleasant, always helpful. She never remarried but raised
two fine and successful children on her own. Praise to
her.

6

Life in Westport

While looking around the Fall River area for a place to live, I found myself on Drift Road in Westport, where I spotted a small "For Sale" sign at the head of a dirt lane that lead to the Westport River. Down to the river I went. In addition to the big old rambling house was the discovery of the remnants of an old stone dock and the figure of a man fishing from a pile of rocks offshore. When I returned with Monny, the fisherman, constructed of driftwood and old clothes, was in the same place. We later named him Captain Seaweed and he stayed there for years until a hurricane took him away.

Monny and I had found just what we wanted: an adventure in living, isolated from crowds on eight acres of land on the river. Our stone dock might have been the same one used by Paul Cuffe. Cuffe was the black Quaker merchant who had built his own ships on our land, sailed up and down the East Coast and became active in the African return movement taking a boatload of freed slaves to Sierra Leone in 1815. Nearby a lane led westward a half mile to the Weiner farm whose current owners were clearly descendents of the Cuffes and Weiners who crewed their own ships. At the head of our lane lived John Roberts with his wife and father. They later became good friends. Since they were black it was possible they had a family connection to Cuffe, but unfortunately we never inquired.

Our discovery at 1504 Drift Road was an old house, a classic handyman's special. The heat came from a single-pipe hot air coal furnace in the cellar with one large opening into the downstairs hall. During our first holiday season, the upstairs became so cold we feared the pipe going up to our only bathroom would freeze. We found an accommodating Ray Hadfield who came immediately and cut a hole in the floor above, thus beginning a long personal and professional friendship.

Later we added an addition to the south that connected to the main house by a small greenhouse. This major wing was to be a library and retreat from my occasionally boisterous and noisy family. The entrance from the outside into the greenhouse connector allowed one to enter the library directly or pass into the main part of the house. In the greenhouse we grew beautiful pink camellias, which I occasionally brought to my patients as they were recovering from surgery. Later, I did the same with the Brownell Tea roses I had planted along the south wall of our property. The patients loved it. I loved it. They would remark to their visitors, "Aren't they beautiful! My surgeon grows them and he brought them in for me." As Dr. Daniel Gallery, my Irish colleague, would say when complimented about his surgical skill, "Tell your friends."

There was also a glassed-in porch on the riverside running the length of the house where Mrs. Baker, the previous owner, had served her famous chicken dinners. For us it became the scene of porch concerts by our three girls with make-believe instruments made from anything lying around the house. Monny and I were excluded until show time when we were summoned to sit enthralled and amused at the "porch concerts."

Monny spent almost all of her time caring for the children and rehabilitating the house. When Mimi and Jay were born, we arranged all the children's bedrooms on the second floor. The stairs led up from the riverside front door. Sue's bedroom was in the southeast corner, complete with canopy bed and a working fireplace. Lucy was next in the southwest corner, a lovely room with built-in beds, carpeting and a Whistler print on the wall. We fit Mimi into a tiny room on the west side with built-in bookcases and slanting ceilings. Judy was in the northwest corner; a room bright with yellow paint, a built-in desk, and her beautiful violin stand in a prominent location. In the northeast corner was Jay's room with a huge blackboard covering one wall. The original bathroom overlooking the river was freshly painted and bright with geraniums in the window. Monny went over every inch of our tired old house, supervising the changes we made, and putting in much physical work herself. Her creative efforts were everywhere.

We gradually settled in to life in Westport. Monny took the girls to the Point for swimming lessons. This was the only time all summer that we let them off the property because of the threat of poliomyelitis. In early June, to celebrate Judy's birthday, we went to Lincoln Park, the nearby amusement park. After that, except for the short swimming lessons, the children were kept at home until Labor Day. Just think. Until the germ theory of disease was established by Pasteur in the 1860's, the cause of almost all disease was unknown and as frightening as polio was in our day.

All our children went barefoot around home with its large yard, the small beach, and a skiff. Occasionally Monny would pile them into the car to get emergency food at the tiny Tripp's Store a mile up the road. After the first few visits we learned that Mr. Tripp, the storekeeper, worried that we did not have enough money for shoes and had considered taking up a collection.

Judy began her life in Westport wearing a football helmet. When she was four years old, she suffered a severe head injury while visiting her grandparents in Hanover, New Hampshire. She was in the front seat when Monny's father, Arthur Barwood, made a slow left turn in front of the Hanover Inn. The passenger door wasn't securely latched and it swung open and Judy partially fell from the car. The door hit an upright granite post and when it slammed back, it caught Judy's head causing a large compound fracture of her skull.

To our good fortune the accident had occurred in Hanover where the quality of medical and surgical care was excellent. I also had a close friend there, Dawson Tyson, who had neurosurgical experience. Also present was the highly qualified neurosurgeon, Henry Heyl. These two men successfully operated on Judy. She was left with an 8 cm skull defect with the expectation of a metal plate closure. She wore the protective football helmet for at least four years with no psychological sequellae. I have a Kodachrome slide of her playing at the Westport Point School with the earflaps of her helmet flopping. She looked like a billy goat. She never needed the plate.

When my day at Truesdale ended and I arrived back in Westport in the evening, I was often asked to make rounds on the girls' dolls. If one suffered from pneumonia, I produced my stethoscope and listened to its chest. If a sore throat was the problem, I carefully used my penlight and looked down its throat. One case was an appendectomy that had been performed that day; it had sutures on its abdomen. I followed that patient regularly until the sutures were removed some twelve days later. The girls, and then Jay and Mimi, often made hospital rounds with me, to the delight of the patients. One time the two small ones sat just outside the operating room while I did an operation.

In our first days in Westport I did not need a telephone answering service because Monny was usually home. If not, a friend of ours, Ruth Howland, presided over the only switchboard in town. If someone called me on our crank up telephone, she would handle the call. Our number was "7 - 5, ring 13." Ruth Howland is still alive in 2004, as kind and gentle as ever.

I went through a convertible phase with a new car every two years. In the winter I rode with the top down, the windows up, the heater on, wearing a cowboy hat. It is a wonder anyone would let this character operate on him. One Saturday afternoon before Easter I was on my way home with the top down on my convertible when I went by a storefront that had a huge white rabbit about six feet tall in the window. I negotiated with the owner, bought it, set it in the seat next to me and brought it home as a present for the family.

We also raised real rabbits starting with two white ones with a small hutch and run for them. During a cold and snowy spell in the winter we paid little attention to the rabbits beyond the necessary feeding. When the weather broke and we opened the hutch to examine them more closely, we found 22 rabbits, white and brown. I have a kodachrome of the rabbits taken in our kitchen where we had let them run loose. The rabbits had grouped themselves by color, white rabbits in one corner, brown rabbits in another. I wonder how Martin Luther King, Jr. would have responded to this natural segregation.

Beagles became a significant part of our activities. One bright morning as I stepped out of the porch there was our mother beagle nuzzling her puppy into the macerated flesh of a freshly caught rabbit. Jay and Mimi were particularly fond of our beagles. When the mother first whelped, Mimi gave up her small bed for the birthing process while she slept on the floor next to the bed. Monny brought beagles to Haiti in a cage on the deck of the freighter that brought her, our two children and all our worldly goods. One time Jay brought a tiny beagle, undetected, to Haiti in his pack or coat pocket.

Monny's vocation was sewing. In her sewing corner in the cellar of the house she made all the lined draperies and curtains for the house, many dresses for herself and the girls, a wool suit for Jay, a luscious red velvet smoking jacket for me, innumerable elaborate Halloween costumes and at least one tutu for Sue. Sewing patterns remain in her room on River Road still, and the closet door is filled with racks of thread. Her technique was meticulous.

Lanz dresses from Boston were a staple of the girls' wardrobe. The shopping trip to Best's or Bonwit's in the big 1880's square brick building across from Brooks was an event. We drove our old green Chevrolet station wagon taking at least an hour and a half, maybe two hours up old Route 138. It seems now like a vignette out of the Victorian age when I write about these excursions. There, upstairs, we all sat on a sofa as the clerk brought out the lovely dresses. We made choices; the girls went back to try them on and then returned to parade before us.

Occasionally our Boston excursions were accompanied by an elegant dinner for the five of us in the high ceilinged, walnut-paneled dining room of the Parker House, one of Boston's oldest hostelries. All the waiters, including the maitre'd, were black and friendly. The headwaiter and Monny had conversations about the fine coffee. He finally divulged their secret. "Madame," he said, "Just use a lot of coffee."

Grateful Jewish patients who either owned or worked in the Fall River shops were a frequent source of clothing for the girls. These folks were very kind to me. We attended their weddings, sedars and bar mitzvahs. Rabbi Samuel Ruderman of the Temple Beth El and his wife Tillie were patients and good friends. B'Nai B'Rith put on an elaborate party for me at the Temple Beth El. Our closest friends in Fall River were Jewish and included the Radovsky family and the jolly Norman Zalkind.

In Westport I caught the antique car bug thanks to my friendship with Allen Pierce and Steve Delano. I purchased a beautiful 1914 Ford Touring car. It was all there except for the acetylene tank on the running board for the headlights. It was bright red with lots of shiny brass. With the windshield down and the cut-out open, we could get forty miles an hour. It was fun while it lasted. At one point we had a small motor-driven racing car that the family put together with Jay. He and Monny took it to the town beach in the station wagon where he could speed around the large paved parking lot to his heart's content.

When Mimi joined the Brownies, Monny became a Brownie leader. One time Mimi wanted to go to Brownie summer camp for a couple of weeks. She and the rest of the troop of fifteen to twenty kids needed a physical examination to qualify for camp. Monny brought them into the clinic and I did a physical exam on all of them. It wasn't a very complicated exam but one that involved eye charts. It was then, to our dismay, that we discovered that Mimi had poor vision in one eye. When the problem was corrected, she discovered she really could see.

When we came to Westport in 1948, we immediately surveyed the community looking for a church where we could worship and bring up our girls. We chose the Westport Monthly Meeting of Friends in Central Village, a modest white building resting between the community house and the town cemetery and facing the St. John's Roman Catholic church and the Grange Hall. Back then it felt more like a Methodist Church than a Quaker meeting despite the sign on the door. We shared the preacher with the Westport Point Methodist Church. The attendance was fairly good but a few of us, and I guess you could say it was the newcomers, wanted the Meeting to become a little more Quakerly. Slowly over the course of several years with support from the kindly Quaker Macomber sisters and without great friction it was transformed to an unprogrammed meeting as it is now. Fifty years later it is blessed with many children and several active young couples. I have never seen it in such good shape. As far as I know, we have never had an unpleasant face-off between individuals or different constituents since 1948. There always seemed to be one or two persons who kept the remnant alive in slender times. I did it for a while with the help of the Macombers. Stewart Kirkaldy did it for a long time as did Lloyd Brightman, and in recent years, Jean Kennison. Now younger folks are carrying on the flame. I don't know how it originated, but early on we had a succession of Harvard Divinity School students coming down to run our worship service. They were wonderful young men and their wives. The first was George Jones, followed by Stanley Johnson whose wedding we attended, Mennonite John Ruth who started our annual book sale, and Edwin and Dorothy Hinshaw who had been young missionaries out in the bush of East Africa. We met them when Monny and I and our two younger children were at Friends Africa Mission in Kaimosi.

Our social life in Westport was low-key. One of our first friends was Dr. Burton Bryan and his wife, Patience. An early event in our association with the Bryans was a dinner party held one winter evening. Our house on the river was a quarter of a mile down a modest hill from the main road. Snow occasionally blocked the driveway so we would leave the car and a sled at the top of the lane. It was a cold night when Pat, monstrously pregnant, got on the sled and barely stopped short of the river.

Our property with its river frontage and wide lawns was perfect for outdoor gatherings. Every year we hosted a picnic for the Department of Surgery which centered around a softball game, beer, soft drinks, and delicious food prepared by Monny. The guests were the surgeons Drs. Atwood, Hawes, Gallery, B. D. Bryan and David Crowell, an anesthesiologist, the two surgical residents, all the O.R. nurses and anyone else who worked there. We swam, went out in the skiff, honed our archery skills with a bow and arrow, played badminton and drank beer. The main event was the softball game where everyone looked ridiculous except the surgical residents. Gallery and others played a lighthearted poker game around our old oak dining room table. The picnic was always a success.

One New Year's Eve we invited Fritz and Ruth Mitchell and Charley and Mary Bryan for a celebration that centered on a roast pig. The Mitchells were affluent supporters of the Truesdale Hospital and close friends of Warren Atwood. Ruth was the daughter of E. P. Charlton, the main supporter of Truesdale's healing initiatives and the hospital. While I was making my weekly consultant rounds at the Newport Naval Hospital I was called to the phone. It was Monny. "I can't get the pig in the oven, it's too long!" We opted to cut it in half. When it appeared on the table that evening Monny had fashioned some kind of wreath around the incision. It was a wonderful party, one I would never attempt now.

On trips to New York, we went to the New York City Ballet and the marvelous musicals of the time. These trips were a major event, glamorized by the mysterious Colonel Rosencranz. Hymen Miller, a manufacturer of children's clothing, was a friend and patient of mine. He and I were talking one day about the theatre and he said, "Oh, gee, Frank, maybe I can get you tickets. I have a friend in New York City whose name is Colonel Rosencranz and I'll be seeing him when I go into New York next week. What would you like to see?" I mentioned one of the current musical hits. In the next week or two he called up, "You're all set, Frank." I replied, "What do you mean?" Miller went on, "Go to the box office about twenty minutes before curtain time and ask for five seats for Colonel Rosencranz and they will have them for you. Pay no money." The three girls, Monny and I headed for New York in the old green station wagon, leaving Westport at 7 o'clock in the morning. We stopped at the home of a friend of Monny's in Bronxville, New York where the girls changed into fancy clothes. In Times Square we grabbed a hot dog, ate it sur la pouce and proceeded with considerable trepidation to the box office. I stepped up to the window, made a show of confidence and said, "You have five tickets for Colonel Rosencranz?" Lo and behold the clerk reached above the window and pulled down five tickets. They were in the twelfth row! It was amazing.

We enjoyed the show immensely and, according to plan, Monny and I took the girls to an elegant restaurant to make up for the hot dog and orange juice we'd had in Times Square. We then drove back home. We repeated this excursion many times often including friends of the girls such as Penny Leuvelink. We saw the first run of shows like *Camelot*, *My Fair Lady*, *The King and I*, *Flower Drum Song*, *I Could See Forever*, and *South Pacific*. Colonel Rosencranz never failed. I eventually paid the standard box office price to Hymen Miller, yet I never learned who Rosencranz was. A mysterious benefactor, he played a significant role in introducing the Lepreau family to the musical theatre world.

On these New York trips, we occasionally stopped at the Bazar Francaise at 666 Sixth Avenue, where Monny purchased nice copper and brass kitchen items. One Christmas she surprised me with all the equipment I'd need for making crepes suzette. The result: the family had weekly crepes suzettes until Monny had mastered the technique of crepe making, and I learned how to be the flashy host without bungling the show. The final product should not be too sweet, not too alcoholic but just right. I pattered on about my finesse, my French father and so on, and kept an essential index card of directions beside me on the table.

In the 1950's Monny and I went for a rare weekend at the Algonquin in New York. There we used Kate Simon's tourist book as our guide, especially the chapter titled "A Night for Insomniacs." We checked in at the Palm Court at Eloise's Plaza Hotel, and maybe the Persian Room at the St. Regis, but mostly we walked the town, rode its busses and its dusty subways. We poked around all-night bookstores, had coffee and pastry in quirky eateries, listened to music of various flavors coming from unseen places.

After the polio scare Monny and I and the three girls made weekly trips to Hyannis Music Circus to see old musicals like *The Student Prince*. We became acquainted with Jim Hawthorne, one of the actors. We have a picture of him in a gilt-laden uniform with the girls, their faces immersed in cotton candy.

At some point in these early years Monny and I and the girls went off to the "undiscovered" Cayman Islands, staying in the small cottage of Mr. Cyril Coe. Grand Cayman was a sleepy place with electricity only four hours a day to keep the dentist's drill running. There was no refrigeration; one bicycled early in the morning to get fresh turtle meat and brought it home tied to the handlebars. One small tourist building stood empty on a beach several miles long. I made rounds throughout the island with a resident from the Jamaican teaching hospital. Hypertension was the most common disease. I did my first overseas surgery on a young woman who had appendicitis. She walked into the operating room and climbed up on the table. I did a spinal, rolled her over, and with a few rusty instruments, saved her from a burdensome trip to Jamaica.

We terminated our planned three-week vacation early. Monny was seven months pregnant with Jay, the heat was oppressive, and we did not appreciate the early calls of the chickens right outside our cottage windows. We'd come to the island sitting amongst assorted freight in an old PBY from World War II, and we left the same way, getting out to the plane in a small boat with a put-put outboard motor. It was an adventure.

Living in Westport, owning property and having children in the local schools, I thought I should do my civic duty. I became active in the parent-teacher association and successfully ran for three four-year terms on the public school committee. When the school committee made an inspection of the school buildings twice a year, I would first go into the basement where the toilets were lined up and flush each one. I found an inordinate number that didn't work. This was an important educational experience for a physician who was used to sitting in his office making pronouncements with patients listening respectfully. In a public office, especially an elected one like the school committee, a physician was treated just like any other ordinary person with no particular prerogatives. That was a great experience for me. I don't know how much good I did but I learned a lot. One lesson in particular was not to make an enemy out of your adversary. Miss Audrey

Tripp was the elementary school supervisor in the old wooden town hall on Main Road. Sometimes she and I disagreed, once because Monny and I wanted our children to have homework and she did not. We had differences of opinion but mutual respect for each other.

Some years later when Miss Tripp had a peptic ulcer, she came to me for surgery. Her ulcer was obstructing the outlet of her stomach, and I knew in such a situation with the surrounding inflammation it would be difficult to get a secure duodenal stump closure, which was mandatory to avoid a fatality. For Miss Tripp and me, it meant emptying her stomach every morning for three or four weeks using a rubber tube. Gradually the inflammation and scarring of the duodenum were reduced, allowing her to eat and improve her nutrition. Her operation and convalescence went smoothly. It was a good thing. If she hadn't made it, I might as well have taken the next bus out of town. Everyone knew Audrey Tripp.

John M. and I were on the Building Committee for a new school and were constantly at each other's throats. One of us wanted twelve classrooms, the other sixteen. I've forgotten the outcome, but I finally realized that John was a rough diamond but an intelligent and good person, and we became friends. A moving experience on the School Committee involved Mike J., a second generation Portuguese. He was an example of the Peter Principle. We had just built the new school and the question arose about naming it. We discussed various names and finally Mike spoke up with a loud, emotional and passionate speech. "I am not smart, just a dumb, ignorant Portuguese. I don't amount to much. But anything good about me or anything that I have accomplished I owe to Alice Macomber. We are going to name that school the Alice A. Macomber School." Obviously we named the school the Alice A. Macomber School. Miss Macomber was a wonderful, old-fashioned Quaker woman who taught in the public schools.

My next community activity brought me in conflict with the old residents and our few friends in the upscale Westport Harbor area. Monny, while buying lobsters at Lee's Wharf at the Point, noted raw sewage running into the river close to the intake for "fresh water" that circulated in the lobster tank. We also noted that when our children swam off our friends' boathouses at Westport Harbor they often developed small boils or pimples, yet the children of the boathouse people did not. Obviously, the Harbor children had developed immunity to the contamination from up the river, or maybe even their own boathouses, which also dumped sewage into the river. My investigation determined that there was much raw sewage emptying into both the East and West branches of the Westport River. I could get no action until I persuaded the state to do something. The state did, and the situation improved, albeit slowly.

When several acres of an orchard abutting our property to the south were suddenly subdivided into small parcels with tiny summerhouses springing up, I quickly became interested in zoning. We feared a trailer park, a gasoline station and all kinds of objectionable activity in our pastoral area. We learned that the few zoning regulations in town were for the most part ineffectual. After much brouhaha, committee meetings, petitions, house calls, controversy and town meetings, we succeeded in updating the zoning regulations. A Catholic lawyer from the north end, an old-time family lawyer from Westport Point and I spearheaded the campaign, and it resulted in the first zoning regulation in town. At that time the town was rather sharply divided between the Catholic north end and the Protestant south end. So it was significant to get this well-known and articulate Catholic lawyer from the north end into the act. There was a body of opposition from certain realtors and others, and strangely enough, the farmers. Their stance was, "This is my land and nobody can tell me what to do with it." Various official town committees and private groups sprang from the zoning law that called for a minimum half-acre lot size and clearly defined residential and business zones.

We gradually became acquainted with many Westporters who became friends. Kay Wood was a lovely first grade school teacher at Westport Point where all our children entered school I had the opportunity to take care of her in later years when she was terribly sick. Her husband, Harold, was an old-time Westporter, tough and square but gentle inside. He was an icon in Westport, a hunter and a fisherman. He had been a football player and a good athlete, and served for many years as the high school principal. The high school auditorium is named after him. I eventually attended him in his fatal illness at home. His family was in constant attendance for the final weeks and I was there much of the time during his last days. It was an emotional and sad experience but at the same time an uplifting one. It was a privilege to be a temporary part of this wonderful family. I was asked to speak at his funeral and used a line from Hamlet, "Good night, sweet Prince, and flights of angels sing thee to thy rest."

Ray Hadfield was considered the best carpenter in the area as well as a good fisherman. He was expensive but good, on time, and reliable. He took me eel lighting one night, an outing that gave me a headache. We got in a skiff with no motor. A bright light on the stern illuminated the river bottom as we passed slowly in water not more than twelve inches deep. As the light illuminated the eels that were moving slowly or not at all on the bottom, we speared them with a metal trident on the end of a lightweight long-handled pole and flipped them into the boat. Later, the eels were skinned, cut into pieces, and dipped in cracker crumbs before frying.

For several years I took my teenage daughters climbing in the Presidential Range of the White Mountains in New Hampshire. We began with Mount Chocorua, a climb that was not too difficult, approaching it from the lake in the foreground with its lovely view. Once on top, the views became wide and spectacular. We climbed Mount Washington several times. A typical trip started out from the Pinkham Notch Camp of the Appalachian Mountain Club where we would spend our first night. The next day we ascended on the Tuckerman's Ravine trail to Lakes of the Clouds. We slept for the night on the shoulder of Mount Washington. We left Lakes in the morning to hike across the peaks with their magnificent views and settle down for a third night at the Madison Huts.

At 6,293 feet, Mount Washington has some of the fiercest weather in the world with conditions that are renowned for changing with amazing rapidity. On one occasion while hiking with Jay, who was ten years old, I lost him in a sudden fog. I could not see the piles of stones fifty feet apart. Occasionally, in summer, a few young people disregard all advice and begin their climb in mid afternoon in the sunshine at the foot of the mountain. Their bodies are found the next day half way up the mountain.

Our climbing experiences were pleasurable and varied. Near the top of Mount Jefferson there is a wide, flat area covered with stones two to three feet in diameter that is called Monticello Lawn. We saw that some wag had placed a lawn mower on it. On one occasion we descended via the long Boots Spur Trail. Poor Judy's quadriceps gave out causing her great distress. A great photograph of Jay and Sue on top of Mount Washington reminds me of our trip to the summit on the cinder laden Cog Railway and the return in rain down the difficult Ammonoosoc Ravine Trail.

As the three older girls approached their high school years, we offered them the opportunity to transfer to a private Quaker-oriented school of their choice. Lucy finished her last two years at the Lincoln School in Providence and went on to graduate from Earlham College in Richmond, Indiana. She became a registered nurse and now practices her profession in Providence, Rhode Island.

Judy, however, turned down our offer, preferring to stay in Westport. She enjoyed her school experience and made long-lasting friendships. Judy also went on to Earlham, continued her interest in Latin and graduated with a concentration in Biology.

Sue, like Lucy, graduated from the Lincoln School. Because she and I were both interested in ballet, we were especially close. While still in high school Suzy spent two summers in New York City studying intensively at the New York City Ballet School under the general supervision of Balanchine, who came occasionally. I watched her a few times, one among many slender young women and girls sweating it out at 85th Street and Broadway in the hot summer without air conditioning, ordered around by strict martinet instructors. When the piano began to play, out they came from the barre, no matter how tired.

Sue went on to the University of Utah because it had a good combination of ballet instruction and academics. She did well. Then she surprised us by eloping with Pat O'Neill. Sue and Pat had two boys, Timothy and Sean, and later their marriage ended in divorce. Sue's life from then on was turbulent. She became extremely interested in athletics, long distance bicycling and swimming. After settling in Wakefield, Rhode Island, near Judy, she attended the University of Rhode Island, majored in Early Childhood Education and graduated first in her department. It continues to remain a paradox that this fit, athletically minded woman, an expert in nutrition, should die of anorexia nervosa at the age of 48. Monny and I did our best. Tormented by grief and indecision we seriously considered bringing her into our household when we returned to Westport. The other children thought taking her in would be unwise. Might that have been the only action that could have pulled her out? Who knows? It was our decision. The disease seemed like a demon with a stranglehold that she couldn't break, a knot around her neck that kept getting tighter and tighter. She couldn't free herself. It was similar to the drug addicts I have worked with who try, but fail to break away from the heroin they know will destroy them. Sue died on October 3, 1993.

My father was with us for less than a year after we moved to Westport. He became seriously ill and for one month we had him in a nice nursing home in Fall River. I saw him frequently, probably daily. He died a respiratory death in 1948. He always coughed a lot and when we studied him in New Haven it was found that he had extensive bronchiectasis.

My mother had a good life in Hastings, where she had many friends. She was a housemother at "Dobbs," the Masters School for Girls in nearby Dobbs Ferry. She subsequently moved to Fall River and had an active life there with many friends. I found good living places for her, but eventually she gave up living on her own and entered Highland Heights, a public housing facility for the elderly and those with physical disabilities. It was the first community social project that Dr. David Greer sponsored and, truthfully, it was due to him that it was ever built. It was a remarkable accomplishment, getting the local community, city, state and federal people working together. It is still functioning. My mother had a fractured hip taken care of satisfactorily by my friend, Dr. James Coleman. Later I was with her when she died of pneumonia at the Truesdale Hospital. She was almost 100 years of age. My parents had always been good to me.

~

As the years went by, I failed to get my physician associates to join in a tightly integrated group. I liked to operate. I was good at it, and I was making quite a bit of money. I told the men to just keep me up there operating and we would split the money equally. It didn't fly.

Perhaps they didn't believe me, thinking I had some angle. Physicians tend to be independent men and women. That is exactly why many of us at that time went into medicine. We valued not being subject to others telling us what to do or giving us a pink slip.

I eventually made the difficult decision to leave Fall River. I had done everything I could surgically in Fall River. At the time the Truesdale Trustees were badgering the medical staff to take on more doctors irrespective of their qualifications. This was anathema to us. I was convinced that the best way to attract quality physicians was through a multidisciplinary integrated group managed with integrity and skill. Therein lay the future of medical practice both for patients and physicians. I thought the new clinic on President Avenue would be a catalyst for a true group, but I was unable to convince my colleagues of any further group activity.

We had lost our resident program and had no affiliation with any other teaching institution. Since I loved to teach, this was a serious loss. I was ready to make a move because I felt I no longer had any special contribution to make in the city. I talked a competent Yale resident, Dr. Phillip Smith, into coming up to work with me and presumably replace me.

Bert Dunphy from the Brigham wrote a piece, *Make a Friend of Your Patient.* And I had done that in my years in Fall River. These patients as friends were hard to leave. We had eight acres and a nice house on the shore of the Westport River. Selling the place is my only regret, not for myself, but for my wife. I didn't realize how much that house and land meant to her. She had put so much personal toil into it. It was not Tara to her but it was that sort of attachment. I finally acknowledged that the old missionary dream was still smoldering.   I recalled that when we were in New Haven, we almost went to Turkey. I must say that my membership in the Religious Society of Friends was a factor. So, I thought, "Let's stop thinking about it and do something." Monny had some reluctance but went along with me on a journey that lasted over fifteen years and took us to East Africa, Haiti, and finally back to the United States and Appalachia.

7

Africa

Where in the world to go and in what setting was a puzzlement. Friends Africa Mission at Kaimosi in Kenya needed a physician to help and relieve Dr. David Hadley and his wife, Ruth, who needed a vacation. So I went to their primitive hospital for the months of September and October 1961. After the first month, Monny, Jay and Mimi joined me. It was an exciting time and a good experience for all of us. But I knew it was not for the long term. Here are a few words from the diary I kept at that time.

September 1, 1961: It was humid and one of the summer's hottest days in New York City when Monny, beat up from the heat, drove into St. Albans Naval Hospital with our green station wagon loaded with unpainted furniture that she was taking home from New York for Jay and Mimi's rooms. She was here to see me off. I was to get a refresher course arranged by Captain Joseph Timmes, Chief of Surgery at this huge Naval Hospital. Joe Timmes was an old friend from the time he was Chief at the Newport Naval Hospital where I consulted and attended surgical rounds on Saturday mornings. He and I performed the first mitral commissurotomy in Rhode Island in the early fifties. It was successful.

September 2, 1961: The London North Airport is like a tired New York City bus station, but the destinations are more exotic. Here at the airport everything was in confusion because of late arrivals. The airport people would not let me go to downtown London because I would not get back in time so I walked around the outskirts and finally took a bus to the new airport terminal on the opposite side of the airfield. Ninety-nine percent of the autos are small and old. The airport was on a busy divided highway and I could see many cars over the hour and a half that I watched from a bench at the bus stop. There was an occasional Cadillac, a few Jags, and one Rolls Royce. The rest were an assortment of old vehicles. The front yards are tiny in this part of town, which is very urban, but all are completely planted with flowers.

Back at the airport waiting area I saw many well-dressed, well-mannered blacks who disappeared just before boarding. I expected them to be on my plane, but as we queued up, no blacks. I departed on South African Airways, an apartheid airline. The blacks that had "disappeared" an hour earlier were on a BOAC prop plane for Nairobi. Ironic for a Friend on a mission like mine to be riding on an apartheid airline.

September 3, 1961: Here in Nairobi. This was a day of luxury, the last one for some time. I stayed at the new Stanley Hotel as guest of the airline. It was lush. I had coffee on the mezzanine overlooking the square at the junction of Delamere and Government Road, the main intersection in Nairobi. That night in my private room, I fell into a sound sleep. At dawn there was a knock on the door, and a black person entered and said something like "tchai". It was the morning tea, a custom in English communities in Africa at daybreak.

I had a swim at the Norfolk Hotel with refreshments at the poolside. The Norfolk, like Shepheard's in Cairo and Raffles in Singapore, was noted among world travelers in Empire days because of the celebrities who stayed there and the stories written about them. Elsbeth Huxley describes the Norfolk in *The Edge of the Rift* and *The Flame Trees of Thika*. From its door, carriages and wagons came and went from the farms in the highlands. We have a *Settlers Cookbook* that gives a good look at life on those farms. The Norfolk itself consists of one large stone building with a big dining room and lounge, and a porch with wicker furniture where we had coffee after the meal. Elegant is the word: lots of beautiful cutlery, china, and all the appurtenances of wealth.

This was Kenya's last year as a British colony. The waiters wore red caps, long white robes with red sashes and they were barefoot. How long would it last? Surrounding the main building were several smooth thatched sleeping cottages and larger luxurious dwellings, also with thatched roofs. Later, after Monny came in October, we had an elegant supper there and I was pleasantly surprised to see three men, one white Englishman, one Indian and one black all well dressed, well mannered eating together in these gracious surroundings. After dinner we went out on the porch and had coffee. It seemed like the heady Empire days, but I doubt if one would have seen then such a mixture of black, white and tan at the same table. There were big game hunters all about. There was a Time Life newsman trying to scoop the National Geographic regarding a new find in the evolution of man near here. Dr. Louis Leakey was blocking him.

September 4, 1961: Up at 5 a.m. To the airport for the plane to Kisumu. Our plane was a twin-engine loaded with freight with a small passenger area. Ruth Hadley met me. We shopped in Kisumu, a town of 27,000 people. First we went to the huge native market where all the produce is on the ground in piles. Small heavy goods are carried on the head. Then to a modern supermarket, smaller than the A & P in Fall River, but with Chicklets, Spry, hot dogs and cake mix all there and presided over by Indian tradesmen. During my whole time in East Africa the businessmen were Indians. In a bank, there was a white manager way in the rear surrounded by a few assistants. The rest were black or Indian. While roaming Kisumu, I saw more Mercedes Benz in a few minutes than I did in London in two hours. All were Indian drivers, presumably owners. It was thirty miles to my destination, Kaimosi, twenty of it over a muddy dirt road. I thought I was into the heart of Africa. Here the women using hoes were doing all the cultivating. Two days ago an African with a bow and arrow had wounded a white woman and her child just ten miles from here. The Mau Mau were moderately active, although not as bad as the year before, and I was told to be wary of them. At the mission I met Fred Reeves, secretary of the mission, and his wife, Inez. They were a wonderful couple, fifty years old, and were leaving for a few days. Friends World Committee, one hundred people here for the weekend, had just left.

Outpatients at Friends Africa Mission sit on a bench along the wall of a long veranda. On my first day as I followed Dr. Hadley down the line he would point out a few patients who had schistosomiasis. "How do you know?" I asked. "A boat just came in from

Tanzania and patients get infected from the lake waters. Here I'll show you." He took a patient into a room off the veranda, put him in the knee chest position, inserted a proctoscope, took a tiny snip of mucosa and put it under an old monocular microscope. There they were: the classic schistosomosis eggs.

Saw all sorts of things at the hospital, which smelled like a stable. Pediatrics was full with 15 patients with malaria, each mother sleeping on the floor beside her child. Others had pneumococcal meningitis diagnosed by smear. There were two cases of meningiococcal meningitis in a male ward with a screen around them. The student nurses got a charge watching me eat their maize, mush and boiled cabbage while sitting on a stool with them. I had a busy day: tonsil and adenoidectomy, salpingogram, pulled two molar teeth, sewed up a flexor tendon of the thumb, treated malaria from a book and did a GI series, which is a fluoroscopy of the esophagus and stomach followed by some x-ray films. Dr. David Hadley did an amazingly skilled and simply done skin graft with four instruments. I finished work at 8 p.m., and then had supper with Dave. He went on to a religious meeting. He and Ruth have a deep, religious faith. I should think one could not carry on in this way very long without it. Dave is here serving God and incidentally man.

September 6, 1961: Dave and Ruth went to Kisumu. Charles Perreira, an ophthalmologist at Presbyterian Hospital in New York City, and I are running the show. I saw many cases of malaria. A patient with Stevens-Johnson syndrome manifested by the usually fatal erythema multiforme is getting better. Made rounds on the whole hospital of one hundred beds.

Had lunch with the Harpers, a couple in their seventies that "retired" here and are now doing the treasurer's work for the mission. They have been all over the world, largely China and the Near East, in missionary and YMCA work. That night had supper with two of the sisters, as the English call their nurses. One teaches in the girls' school and the other in a teacher's training school. One has strong anti-Zionist and anti-British sentiments. At 7 p.m. Dr. Perreira and I led a worship service at which I was introduced and asked to say something, but as usual, I was not articulate in matters of religion.

September 7, 1961: At 7 a.m. I walked to the sawmill and power station where I took pictures. Dr. Hadley is a driver in a mild unassuming way. He keeps moving and makes all decisions rapidly and acts upon them. By "driver," I don't mean that he drives others; Dr. Hadley drives himself and carries everyone with him.

More outpatients today. I did three skin graft dressings for Dr. Hadley with remarkably good results, given the environment in which they were done. There were flies all over and the mother and aunt were looking over my shoulder. Just finished at 6 p.m. when Dr. Hadley disappeared to deliver a baby, then supper, then a staff meeting.

September 8, 1961: Busy, busy, 7:30 a.m. to 11 p.m. Did a bilateral femoral hernia with me on one side, Dr. Hadley on the other. Did a vagotomy and pyloroplasty, which was easy on a slender female. They are all thin out here because there is not enough food, usually one meal a day of pouche. I think "pouche" is made from some kind of grain, perhaps corn and beans. Did a cystoscopy, pulled a molar tooth, many outpatient cases, usually tapeworms, hookworms, schistosomiasis, ascaris, malaria and the like. I did two cesarean sections, one for an all-night prolonged labor. Both were extremely ill patients who had taken African medicine to strengthen labor contractions. In one, the child was stuck in the mid pelvis, pulse of 155, blood pressure 90 when we began. I made a short transverse incision in the uterus that was too low but I was able to get it together. No blood transfusions available. Mother and child doing well today.

September 9, 1961: Full day again. Pulled two teeth, a cysto, sigmoidoscopy, bronchogram, D&C. Lunch with two nurses, dinner with Oscar and Olive Marshburn. Dr. Hadley played a Chopin piece on the piano. Saw slides of Murchison Falls and lots of game. Wonderful to hear from Monny today. Asked her to come out. Tomorrow at 4:30 a.m. I will be up to hear the drums beat.

The most significant event since I have been here was a hospital staff meeting where important decisions were made by Quaker consensus. Many decisions involved sensitive issues such as holiday time, living conditions, family, policies, salaries and personalities throughout the hospital. Dr. Hadley, a perfect clerk, felt that the Mission should gradually pass all the activities to the Africans as soon as they can handle it. The lack of facilities is appalling. Not a single x-ray therapy machine available in all of East Africa.

September 10, 1961: Lots of church. Up at 4:30 a.m. to hear African drummers and chant. Meeting at 11:15. Meeting again at 6:15. We sang, *Follow the Master*, a beautiful hymn. Later at Fred Reeve's house, we saw his African movies and slides which included one of a rope with white hands sliding off to give way to the black African hands. Fred Reeve, an amazing man and an ex-contractor, has been here since 1954 except for two years on leave. Built all kinds of things since coming.

September 11, 1961: Kisumu most of the day with Ruth Hadley. Had mutton curry at the Rendezvous, which is an arm of King's Inn Hotel. It was good. Tried without success to photograph three Indian schoolgirls in green tunics and loose white pants. The Indians run Kisumu and much of East Africa. All the shops, maybe the banks and the Mercedes are theirs. They are handsome; males and females look just like Europeans except for their color. Some of the older ones are particularly impressive with white beards and hair. At a market I saw a woman smoking a cigarette with the burning end in her mouth. Bought some books in an East African library.

I helped Dr. Hadley do a pyloroplasty, vagotomy and a gastrostomy. We had one retractor. He cut into the vena cava, but we got it patched and all is well. Hadley has a great sang-froid. I did a ureteral transplant into the bladder following an old injury from a hysterectomy. The patient had a ureteral vaginal fistula. She was always dripping urine without control and always wet, a tragic but frequent complication of childbirth in underdeveloped countries. The procedure went slowly but well, two African nurses helping with few instruments. I broke one of the only Foley's catheters they had out here and let out a loud "God damn" which surprised and shamed me in this holy air.

The nurses all have morning prayers. Dr. Hadley reads aloud two pages of "Christian Perfection" by Fenelon each morning at breakfast. He and wife Ruth pray extensively at breakfast each morning. Biopsied a neck node without retractors, without assistance, without ties, excised a femoral node similarly, aspirated a knee plus a full day in the operating room. Dr. Hadley taking x-rays and seeing outpatients all day.

This night while I was at the Reeves' house about 10:00 p.m., we heard a lot of noise like crying. He flew out of the house and into the car with me and drove at full speed up the muddy road with the search light on, to the Bible Institute, where he said the noise came from. He found a bunch of screaming women who thought the noise was coming from Mission Hill. Up we went into the deep woods, into the bushes totally unarmed. He showed absolutely no fear. He walked fast, aggressive like a typical movie detective. I was impressed and scared. He obviously was not. We found nil. He said later it is better not to show evidence of fear at any time. On a similar occasion he cornered and disarmed an African armed with a machete. I think in Kenya it was called a ponga.

September 13, 1961: Dr. Hadley left me alone at the hospital. Nathan, the African medical assistant, steered me through the complexities of tropical disease and medications. When I went off to lunch with Sister Mabel and Irene he ministered to the remainder. I had a clinic of 25 people, most of them with malaria. We have an established case of tetanus. He is having intermittent spasms. He is in constant opisthotonos, almost rigid with frequent spasms all over. We snowed him with one gram of phenobarbitol and 1000 cc of saline drip with two and a half percent pentothol available nearby if he has real trouble. He is an awfully nice, well-spoken, handsome young man. 50% mortality in these cases.

For lunch I had a curry with Mabel and Irene. The former is an American who had been doing missionary service in the Congo. Irene is quite English, reserved, always has tea in spite of all else. She is heading for a leave to Mombasa and the Indian Ocean beaches. I can hardly wait for Monny to come. Prayer meeting tonight and I find that I am "it" next week. I feel like a heathen amongst these missionaries. They look like such good Christians and I am not. I haven't the slightest idea of what I will talk about.

September 14, 1961: Interview tonight with Dr. Whittaker, a government radiologist at King George VI Hospital in Nairobi. He is the only radiologist for this 1,000-bed hospital, 150 beds for active tuberculosis, 80 beds for orthopedics. He says most of the beds are active and if a patient stays more than a month, a hospital staff committee wants to know why. All the funds for the hospital are generated within Kenya, including maintenance of the plant and salaried positions. They are extraordinarily short staffed. He says they have two physicians. Besides the one radiologist at King George VI Hospital, there may be four other x-ray men in Kenya some place.

The following are some notes on the medical school. Mr. Ted Gratten (King George VI, P.O.Box 30024, Nairobi) is the one to see about medical school. There is a meeting this week in Kampala, Uganda with representatives of the East African University and others interested in discussions involving the medical school. Mr. Gratten, a thoracic surgeon, is much interested in getting it started. The hospital facilities at Kampala are saturated now, and it would seem that a new unit in Nairobi is more feasible than increasing the size of

Makerere in Kampala. But where is the money and the staff coming from, particularly when independence arrives? Informal polls indicate that practically all the European staffs of the districts and many at King George VI Hospital might leave with independence. The one thing that might keep them would be the establishment of a medical school at Nairobi. There is already one engineering branch of the university.

The medical ability of the African graduates from Makerere is excellent, equal to that of any English medical school graduate, but their ethics and morals are not. I visited Makerere Medical School and the Mulago Hospital, two of the world's finest tropical medical centers and associated with the London School of Tropical Medicine. Amin later ravaged them. Dennis Burkett who had begun as a solo medical missionary, wrote his Burkett's Lymphoma papers from here and also his other major observation noting the low roughage western diet as a contributing cause of colon cancer and diverticulitis.

In Nairobi, private practice is cash first at seven shillings, exam quickly by an M.D., and treatment by "dresser." There are no house calls. King George VI is a government hospital, no private practice allowed. Aga Kahn Hospital has its own staff, no private practice allowed. A European Hospital is like an English nursing home. Private patients go there, but no Africans allowed on the staff. Dr. Whittaker does not like it

October 6, 1961: Monny arrived in Kisumu with the two children, but no one was there to meet her. A car from the Kaimosi mission 30 miles away happened to be in town and saw a white woman with two small children wandering around and picked them up. It was a cold rainy evening when they appeared at my stone house. We huddled around a small stove, ate some cheese and crackers and hot tea — quite a change from her beginning several thousand miles away in Westport. For my birthday she brought a recording of *Mac the Knife*.

We had a wonderful luncheon with Roger and Mrs. Carter, English Friends, nice house, nice effect, with some oil paintings. Good talk. They spent three and a half years in the States. He is attached to the English education system in England and has been here a year as a Principal at the Teacher Training College. No Englishman here knew any product of Summerhill, an English school using a unique teaching technique that had intrigued me.

October 15, 1961: Great day, busy at the hospital in the morning. Trying to get finished so I can have a half day off that the sisters gave me, but still left some patients sitting on the verandah. "Always one more standing in line". Went with Oscar Marshburn and Tom Lungho to Mbale Monthly Meeting. A great experience: four hundred people; elders in front, Monny, me, Oscar and Tom on the "platform". A buxom female singer dressed in white made us all sing. Oscar gave his usual fine address. Afterward, at lunch, we had rice, chicken, sauce, butter sandwiches and delicious tea. An African custom: in one hand the host carries a towel and a kettle of warm water which he pours over your hands, collecting the water in a bowl in the other hand which contains a bar of soap.

I had a good visit to Chevakali, an excellent high school financed by I.C.A., Kaimosi, Earlham College in Indiana and local money. It was well equipped, with good discipline, eager students, many who walk five to ten miles a day to and from the school. Mr. Kirk, the headmaster, was principal of Barnesville for eight years just before coming. He had one year at a big Youngstown, Ohio high school where he was guidance counselor. Says he doesn't know about native intelligence because there are no good tests. For teachers, a four-year contract is required or two times two years. The transportation is paid. Three thousand dollars a year, excellent equipment, good staff.

I went by myself from Kaimosi to Nairobi for a weekend on a standard African bus overflowing with people, automobile tires, produce, and innumerable personal effects. Once seated I was fixed. My seat was next to a pregnant woman with morning sickness. I stayed at the modern new Stanley Hotel located at the corner of Government and Delamere Roads, the center of the city. Sitting on the corner in an outdoor café I had black coffee and watched the world go by. And indeed it did, in this final year of Kenya as a British colony. Everything was working and peaceful. I was breathing the air of the Empire that was to pass in a few months.

On leaving the next day the station platform was bedlam, swarming with people of multiple colors and languages. A blackboard on the platform showed passengers' names for first and second-class. Only two names were listed for first class: both white Europeans. The evening train back to Kisumu even enhanced my illusions. The corridor was on the side with openings into the compartments where I could see Indians cooking their meals. I had a pleasant visit with a sophisticated black African Mennonite preacher. The dining car and its furnishings seemed left over from the Victorian era. There were side lamps at the windows, tables for two or four covered with white cloth and shining silver. There was a man in military uniform and a typical English settler in shorts, knee-length stockings and brogues. Of course the black waiters wore long white robes and red fezzes.

The old coal firebox of the engine had been converted to oil and one could see the fire as the train took a curve. The vegetation on the right of way was floodlit so passengers could see any animals. I saw none. I slept little because I was entranced by the novelty. I wanted to be awake as we crossed the Rift, see the early morning mist, the wide green views, and the rising sun. Livingston, where are you?

October 16, 1961: I had a visit from the Radleys from South Africa, where he was Head Master of Ashworth Friends School, now on their way home. They had been in South Africa for three years. He gave a historical account and a description of the present situation. The burden of his talk was that the Dutch came into the Cape when only Bushmen and Hottentots were there, then Bantu came from the north beginning in the 1730's. The English came last and settled in the Cape and Natal. The Boers wanted to be alone and moved north to be by themselves. If they could see the smoke from another chimney then that was too close. French Huguenots came as a result of persecution at home.

October 19th will be an election in South Africa in which one million people will vote on the way Apartheid will be administered in the country, particularly toward ten million Africans: 1,500,000 colored, 500,000 Asians, none of whom have a vote. Also there is a great schism between the British and Afrikaner.

October 18, 1961: Bob Mills, the Mission agricultural man, is down feeding the Masai who usually live on blood and milk from the same cows. They have a way of drawing the blood from the neck of the cow, stopping it, then mixing it with milk. The Masai are starving by the thousands. Bob Mills and the others are taking food to them. Otherwise, the Masai men would not know how to cook it and would convert it all to liquor and drink it up before they get home.

Plastic surgery all day. A woman with large holes in her ears wanted them closed so she could become a Christian. Achieved a good result. Finished at 6:15 p.m.

Oscar and Olive Marshburn:

Let not your doubt betray you lest you lose the good you might do by fearing to make an attempt.

John G. Whittier:

Early hath life's mighty questions stirred within the heart of youth. With a deep and strong beseeching what and where is truth?

October 22, 1961: TB rounds before I left, as well as rounds on all patients. Worship service at 9:15 when I spoke briefly about being grateful of the opening that led me to come and see the great work the staff was doing under God's guidance. I don't think I could have handled a month alone without Nathan, the African medical assistant. Beatrice of midwife fame, came to say good-bye at the house with ten eggs, a meaningful and significant gift. They all floated which, I think, means they were over age.

Fred and Inez Reeves drove us down to the boat at Kisumu. There, waiting at Hippo Point on the shores of Lake Victoria, were Irving and Gladys Parker and Alfred and Enola Henderson who were having a picnic supper with the sun setting over the Kovorando Gulf and a full moon coming up on the other side of the sky. They remained standing on the dock waving until we could barely see them.

The terms of working at Kaimosi Hospital: $2,500 plus three quarters of medical bills, tuition for all children, I think that is what he said. A four-year contract. Move all effects out. Housing and light are supplied, and I think a yardman, too. Very tempting. I think most of the group is going to stay. The Parkers go December 31st. Wonderful, wonderful people. It was a little tear jerking to leave them all.

I learned more about Oscar Marshburn. In 1917 at age 21 and married just one week, he went to France to work with Rufus Jones and the newly founded American Friends Service Committee. Oscar and his wife, Olive, were wonderful people. He had a gift for speaking, but mostly he and his wife were doers-doers. He organized the pharmacy, and Olive spent almost all the day playing with the African children. Well into their seventies, the Marshburns were sweet people – a credit to any religious persuasion. I am glad they are Quakers. They made us look good.

October 23, 1961: Nice ride to Port Bell. The moon was out showing a big mountain on the left of the Gulf as we slid out. All third class passengers are up in front sleeping in one long bunkroom. I am not sure whether

men are segregated or not. A few second-class and more
first class passengers were on the upper deck in the
saloon. We were with Asians in a small outside cabin.
We had an OK trip. Port Bell and Kampala were pretty.
The latter is on seven hills. Saw the lovely new Mulago
Hospital. United Touring got us a Morris Minor car, and
two third-class African bus tickets back to Nairobi.

Onward to Masindi, the Victoria Nile and our
destination at the Para Lodge overlooking the river. It
was a long ride in our tiny car through tall grass,
woodlands and African wildlife to Masindi, but soon we
were at the edge of the river where we were invited onto
a raft of few planks for the car wheels and a small area to
stand. It was powered by a small put-put. I have a photo
of Mimi surveying our transport. We crossed about a
mile below the spectacular Murchison Falls, where the
mighty Nile roars through a twenty-foot opening
contained on both sides by tall stone cliffs and then drops
130 feet. Later we were to see it up close via a launch.

At Para Lodge, we elected to stay in the tents. We
had two, each one furnished with two cots, a washstand,
washbowl, and pitcher of water. Each tent was covered
with mosquito netting and on top of that a canvas to keep
us dry. Monny decided to sleep in one tent with one
child and I slept with one in the other tent. As the night
wore on, one of us called in a hoarse whisper, "Frank?"
or it might have been "Monny?" The other was wide-
awake. So we got up, went out and sat in the directors
chairs. She opened her suitcase, where she had kept a
bottle of sherry locked up for a month while we were at
Friends African Mission. We uncorked it and sat there in
the moonlight overlooking the glistening Nile River. The
sounds of the jungle and the heads of the hippos popping

up and down in the river entranced us. It was quite
romantic.   We eventually went to bed, but at dawn
Monny was terribly frightened because she thought an
elephant trunk was coming through the flaps in the tent.
It was an African attendant who was bringing her
morning tchai or morning tea, which was standard in
British Africa.

Para Lodge was magnificent.   Dinner was at 8:00
p.m. with coffee served later in the lounge that
overlooked the river. We first watched a beautiful sunset
over the Nile with the Ruwenzori Mountains in the
background. Bright moonlight followed the sunset. What
a sight!   At dinner there was a potpourri of people
including Bunny Watts, a prosperous, thin 55-year-old
settler from Tanzania who knew all about game habits.
The next day he went on our launch trip and made it an
adventure. Watts looks like the movie version of a thin,
debonair, carefree and sophisticated yet very gay well-to-
do ranchman, which he is.   He races horses and knows a
hundred stories.   Also there was a South African who
came up to Tanzania eight years ago and has become a
successful farmer.   He looks like the typical farmer.   The
next day Kingsley Heath, a noted white hunter, appeared
after three months in the hospital recovering from a lion
mauling.

The following morning we were taken in a launch
up the Nile fairly close to Murchison Falls where the
river rushes through the 20 foot wide cleft. The river was
congested with hippos. You could put your hand over
the side and pat them on the nose as they went up and
down. Nobody seemed apprehensive so we weren't
either.   On the shore there were big crocodiles, sinister
looking with their mouths wide open.   Little white birds

were in their mouths, cleaning their teeth. These crocodiles are dangerous: if they catch you, they take you down to the bottom of the river until you get nice and soft and rotten, and then they take care of you. I photographed all kinds of other animals including elephants, coming down to the shore.

Subsequently, in our little Morris Minor, we toured the countryside with explicit directions to stay away from elephants and to be back on time. We intended to follow those directions, yet at one point, we were steaming around a corner and found ourselves in the midst of them. There was a huge male elephant standing on an elevated bank at the edge of the road. He appeared to be the master of a herd of 20 or 30 elephants that went marching in single file across the road ahead. We stopped. Nothing untoward happened but somehow one of the animals took an interest in us and we had to get away fast. I have a picture taken from the back window of that elephant chasing us. As we drove along, the park became wilder by the minute. Suddenly a crowd of baboons jumped down on the car. I was driving fast and they scattered.

On another trip we were lost at dusk in an electrical storm: rain, thunder and lightening on the shores of Lake Albert. Lake Albert is the boundary between Uganda and the Congo. We were indeed in the heart of Africa, the literary land of Vachel Lindsay and Joseph Conrad. More realistically it was the land of the intrepid explorers. Baker, Burton, Speke and Grant, all looking for the source of the Nile, and Stanley looking for Livingstone. We were far off base on an overgrown track in the high grass when, suddenly, there in the lights of our little Morris Minor containing Monny and me and two little children, was a real lion. I don't know how we got out of that confrontation with the lion, but nothing happened. Mr. Wolfenden, the manager of the lodge, told us we were stupid. One should give the elephants a wide berth as they can run 35 mph, overturn a car and sit on it. We called the episode "Monny and her elephants."

We left Kampala in a third-class African bus with the driver's foot to the floor, charging across Central Africa, careening around curves, and honking incessantly. Mimi and I shared a seat with a large African Muslim lady who said her beads constantly over Mimi who slept in her lap.

October 27, 1961: Nairobi after seven days doing the parks. Met Allen and Mary Bradley, the Head Master of Kamuasinga, and Pearl Spoon, and lunched with them. Again all are urging us to stay. They have two sons in England who like it in Africa and feel this is home. The school year began in January. Kamusinga will be the third largest school in Kenya. It will become one of the few that prepare in Science and Humanities. Went into the African locations with them to the Friends Center, which has many-sided support, but under the aegis of the Friends Service Council of London. It is a busy active place in the midst of slums.

October 28, 1961: The Queen's Hotel was nice, if a bit crowded, with four in a small room but with a large verandah overlooking the street. Morning tea came at 5:45 a.m. after a poor night's sleep because I kept fretting about airline reservations. I called Mr. Loewenthal, the manager, at home at 7:00 a.m. He gave me the name of his uncle in Jewish Jerusalem, a lawyer, Mr. Alfonse Lowenthal, House Freund, Beth Hakeral, Jerusalem. By

8:30 a.m., we had decided to go on an 11:00 a.m. plane altogether to Cairo and Jerusalem, to Tel Aviv and Monny to spend a day in Greece, and me another day in Israel.

Walter Martin met me at the bank with one thousand shillings, the equivalent of $150. He came here five years ago, the first Quaker worker in Nairobi, and started the Friends Center. He was there for five years. Now he is the executive secretary of all Friends activities in Nairobi. He tells me the same story as always with great modesty. He often becomes engulfed by the magnitude of the task and the seemingly insurmountable problems great and small. Sometimes he feels he is making no contribution at all, but must keep going largely on faith. He mentioned that one must be able to accommodate without sacrificing basic principles. Where is the middle ground?

The Friends School in Ramallah on the West Bank was our base. The staff was generous with time and information and definitely pro-Arab. Not long afterward in one of the recurring crises, Lloyd Brightman of Westport Monthly Meeting replaced the headmaster. His calm demeanor cooled the air.

We went to meeting and saw all the usual sites including the Garden Tomb near a wine press, as the Bible says, in the garden of a rich man. It is also known as the Place of the Skull because across a vale some natural excavations in a cliff resemble a skull. British General Charles "Chinese" Gordon, a Bible student, called attention to it in 1882 when he was stationed in Palestine. The tomb is of white stone with places for three bodies and a fourth unfinished crypt. On the ground in front is a small stone trough to accept the large stone disk at the site, which can be rolled over to close the tomb.

On another day we were in the other tomb where Jesus was laid out, now the centerpiece of the imposing Greek Orthodox Church of the Holy Sepulcher. Apparently Jesus was a wandering corpse. Later, I could stand on huge stones of the most holy Via Dolorosa where Jesus carried the cross and without moving my feet, could see something sacred to Judaism, the Dome of the Rock where Mohammed rose to heaven and soldiers walking the walls with Tommy guns. The main street in Nazareth was too narrow for cars. There were buildings on both sides, and what seemed like an open sewer running down the middle. Thence on foot to Israel. From the shore of the Dead Sea we walked uphill across a blistering desert towards the caves where the scrolls were found. Too hot, we turned back. The road passing from Jordan into Israel was tortuous and marked by pylons. None of us could walk across the line into Israel and return to Jordan, so we had to push our suitcases across the line first.

In Israel, our host was the sister of our good friend Rabbi Ruderman of Fall River, and her family. They had gone into Haifa in 1948. As we talked in the living room their 13-year-old daughter said she was going on a hike on the coming weekend. I asked her to elaborate and she described a fifty-mile walk with a full military pack. There in Israel we did all the sites, ate lunch bedside the Sea of Galilee, saw carp farms and Tiberius. The Holy Land adventure was exciting, full of paradox and questions, and I recommend it to anyone. I cannot recall details without notes, but my snap conclusions after a few days with good people on both sides of the Israel/Jordan line are:

1. The enmity and distrust of the two is deep.
2. Israel is clean, green and prosperous.
3. Jordan is dirty, brown and poor.
4. Official policy is often bypassed to make life work. For example, there is no official way to fly from an Arab country into Israel. So I buy a ticket in Jordan to Beirut, but my plane lands in Tel Aviv.
5. A search for the origins of Christianity is obscured by mythology and the modification or fabrication of events to support a belief.

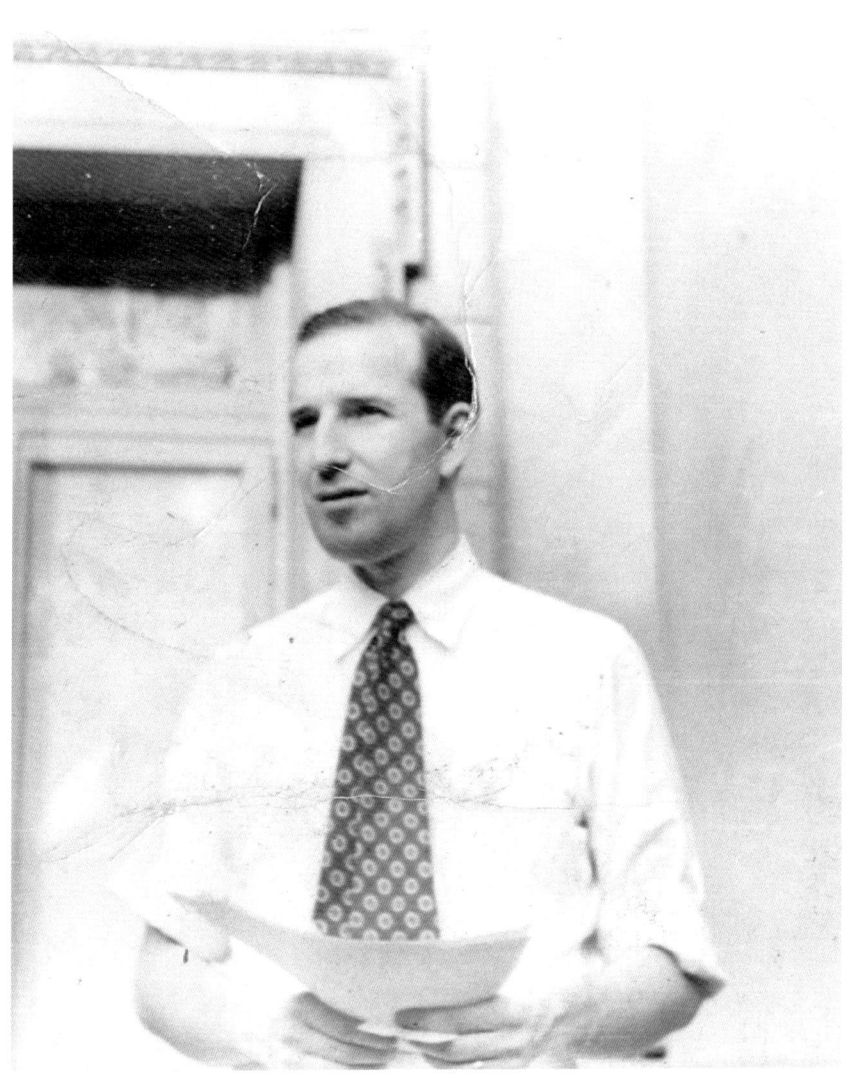

Resident Surgeon at Yale-New Haven Hospital

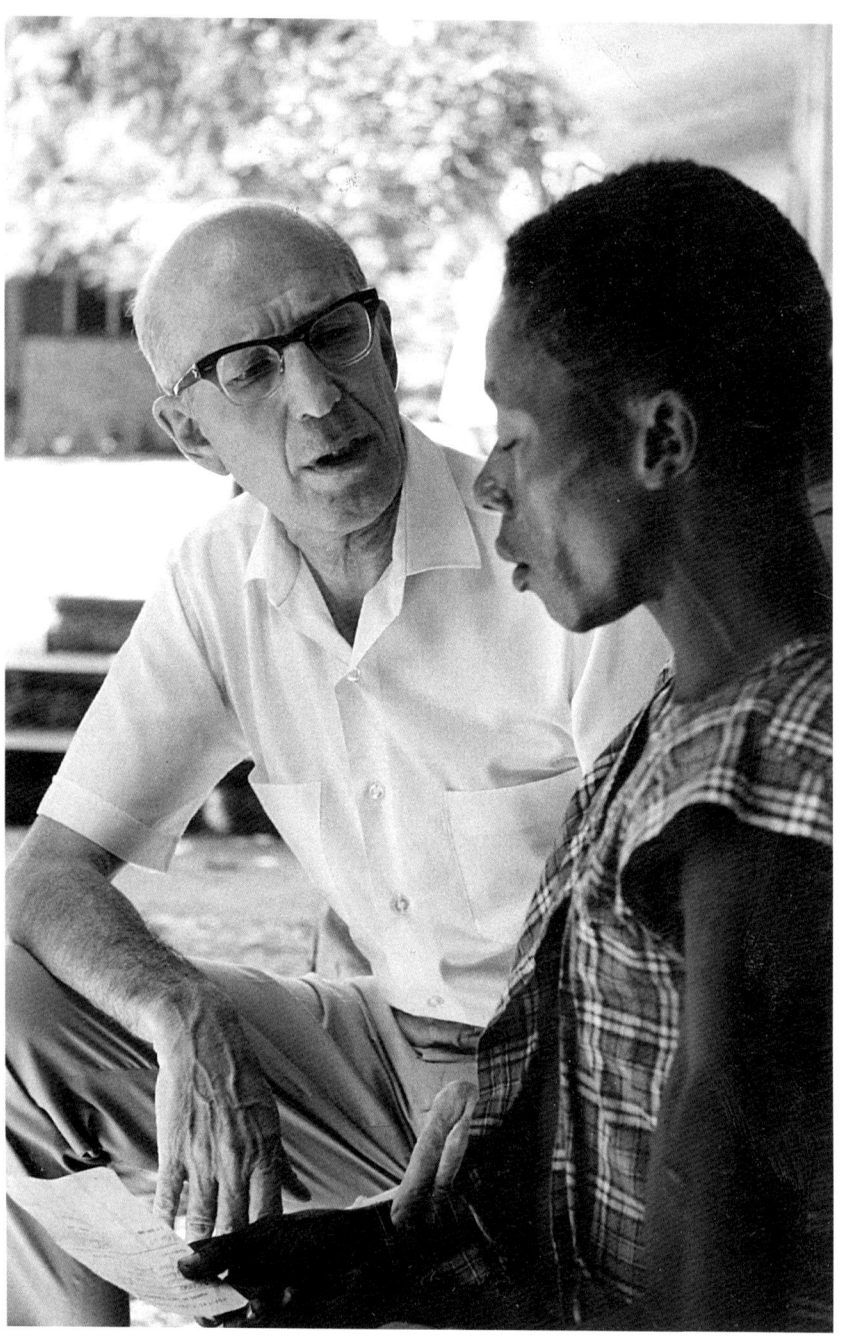

With Patient in Haiti

8

Haiti – a Professional Endeavor

After my brief time at the Friends Africa Mission, I was open to other opportunities to use my medical and surgical skills in an undeveloped country. During a weekend at Tanglewood, Clee Dodge Rea, the husband of Kenny Rea, Monny's best friend at Wellesley, called my attention to Hôpital Albert Schweitzer in Haiti. I traveled to Haiti for a one-month tour in 1962 and again in 1963. Considerable soul searching preceded our decision to commit to a full-time, eighteen-month tour in 1964. About the first of July of that year, I left Monny in Westport to pack up the house, rent it out, and join me. She arrived within a few months with Mimi, Jay, and our beagles, Scott, Keats, and Bulldozer. I have wondered how Monny would have reacted had she known then that we would be in Haiti for almost ten years.

The Schweitzer Hospital had been founded and funded by W. Larimer (Larry) Mellon. At age 37, he decided he wanted to follow the example of Dr. Albert Schweitzer. He received his medical training at Tulane University in New Orleans. Once the hospital was set up in Haiti, however, he did little medical work. He was out of doors working in community development, particularly searching for springs in the hills surrounding the valley and then, surveying and laying pipe into the village to bring a constant source of fresh water. When we were together he would introduce me thus, "Dr.

Lepreau is the inside man, I am the outside man." Our philosophy, carved in the cement slab over the doorway, was Schweitzer's "Reverence for Life".

Dr. Mellon's devoted wife, Gwen, was intensely loyal to his lifestyles, whims and mission. She was tall and attractive with high cheekbones and a commanding presence. She had graduated from Shipley Girls School in Philadelphia and from Smith College in 1934, the same year I graduated from Dartmouth, and was always in the higher social circles of the East. Once she told me how she and her contemporary, Doris Havemyer, roller-skated amongst the Renoirs and Cezannes in the Havemyers' apartment. When she met Dr. Mellon, she became a cowgirl in the Southwest before moving to a nice house and the social scene in New Orleans, where she studied to be a laboratory technician while her husband went to medical school.

Gwen had boundless energy and considerable manual dexterity with pottery, sewing and metalworking. If she put her mind to it and had an appropriate manual, I am sure she could have accomplished major repairs on the large turbines at the hospital. With her superior intelligence, her sensitivity to personalities, and her fluency in English, French, and Creole, she was the perfect one to preside over the daily activities of Hôpital Albert Schweitzer. But always, like everyone else, her projects were subject to Dr. Mellon's approval.

Working at the Hôpital Albert Schweitzer was a tremendous experience with wonderful colleagues, both Haitian and foreign, all united in one purpose: to heal the sick with compassion. Dr. Mellon was a knowledgeable and broad-minded chief who expected quality performance. Gwen Mellon's lieutenants were Miss Pete in Nursing, Boss Andre in the machine shop, Gerard de Vastey in the business office, Mr. Angus in housing and myself in medicine. The international medical staff of men and women consisted of three physicians in medicine, three in surgery, three in pediatrics, one ophthalmologist, one dentist and one anesthesiologist.

Gwen and I had a fine working relationship. Three days a week she worked a full day in the hot steamy clinics as an interpreter and assistant to the physicians. Even though she could be responsible for a doctor's being moved around or out the next weekend, she never interfered with medical decisions.

The panoply of people, disease and culture at Hôpital Albert Schweitzer presented a new mixture every day. The physical facilities at the hospital were good and living conditions were reasonable for my wife. The climate was varied: hot and dry for six months and rainy for the other six, when everything became moldy. Mornings, however, were always clear.

I made an official trip to Grand Riviere Du Nord, within a few months of arriving, to visit a small Mennonite hospital and to see about sending tuberculoses patients to Schweitzer if they could be helped by surgery. Monny and I went with Hyance, the driver, in the hospital Land Rover to Gonaives, to Cape Haitien and to Grand Riviere. Our hosts were Dr. and Mrs. Paul Derstine, the Mennonite head of the unit. It was a friendly visit. All the meat we ate had been canned in Kansas. It was raining and cold most of the time. The roads were covered with water both coming and going. The place was primitive and the entrance to the hospital looked like Hospital Street at Lambarene. They had one case of full-blown tetanus.

After this initial trip, we saw little of the country, as I did not want to be distracted from my purpose in coming to Haiti. I was there to heal the sick. I immersed myself in the hospital and its personnel. Monny and the children and I rapidly became part of the hospital community, both Haitian and foreign. After a year or so I was put on the Board of Directors of the Grant Foundation. I thought this was where we would make policy, but of course the "we" was Dr. Mellon.

After being in Haiti for six months, I could say that everything was going well. We had Saturday morning clinical meetings, which were a great success, particularly because the medical men were outstanding: Rene St. Leger, Gerard Smarth and Francois Charles. Dr. Gerard Frederique, our ophthalmologist, added spice. The Saturday morning meetings, according to Arthur Bergner, a visiting medical student, resembled being at a Massachusetts General Hospital conference. We had the proceedings typed up, bound, and presented to Dr. Mellon as a Christmas gift the first year I was there. Discipline in the medical staff was not a problem for me. All the doctors loved their work, some so much that I occasionally told them to take it easy. I rarely brought a personnel problem to Dr. Mellon for I knew what his response would be. The threat was rarely exercised, but always there: "Well, Frank, there is a car going to Port in the morning and perhaps he could be on it." That meant the person was fired and must leave the country.

Our feeling of being overwhelmed by the workload was lightened by social events of our own making. I recall a dinner party for the staff at the

Mellons' house, which I had arranged. I talked Monny and Gwen into being the waitresses. They dressed up in Ternette heavy blue gingham dresses and went barefoot. They were not allowed to speak, but they were to wait on us. We had a great time. The piece de resistance was Dr. Mellon at one end of the table and I at the other, making crepe suzettes.

The Haitian dictator "Papa Doc" was indeed ruthless. Doctor Francois Duvalier came to power (1957 – 1971) because he led a successful United Nations program to eliminate the dreadful disfiguring disease, yaws, by giving everyone a shot of penicillin. We experienced his cold-bloodedness first hand when a Haitian family who lived on our grounds at Deschapelle was visited one night. There were some gunshots. The building was emptied and remained so until it became the base for our public health activity.   He and his regime seemed to know everything. My family and I had been in Haiti about two months when Dr. Mellon and I were "invited" to a reception at the Palace in Port-au-Prince. We were standing around when a white man came up, said hello to Dr. Mellon and me, saying, "I am Dr. Laughlin." Dr. Mellon replied, "I want you to meet Dr. Lepreau, our new medical director." Dr. Laughlin replied, "Oh, yes. Fall River, isn't it? How are your wife and children?"

One day I was at my dentist in Port-au-Prince when he told me, between filling my cavities, that Papa Doc's men had filled the house across the street the previous night, doing away with the whole family, small children to grandma.   Duvalier's secret police, the dreaded Ton Ton Macoutes, were everywhere.   My instructions, nay, my *orders* to new staff were "Don't even *think* Haitian politics. I had a Ton Ton as a grateful patient who occasionally brought Monny a heart of palm. It made me nervous. When Baby Doc took over, things were a bit looser and this particular Ton Ton went out of town in one of our vehicles under a peach basket. As is usual with a dictator, the country ran smoothly. Monny, a small, white woman, fearlessly walked the streets of Port-au-Prince at night, unmolested.

The Artibonite Valley was lush and green six months of the year because of the rain that fell every afternoon in Haiti, but during the dry season the land was brown and the canals were choked with grass and dirt. Life gave little evidence of the twentieth century. Machetes and long-handled, heavy hoes were the only tools available for coaxing vegetation from the rocky land; cornmeal was pounded out in hollow tree trunks; rice was winnowed by young children running barefoot through it. In the nine years I was there I did not see a piece of farm machinery drawn by either animal or tractor. Precisely because it was underdeveloped, Dr. Mellon chose the Artibonite Valley as the site of his modern, 133-bed hospital. There were major difficulties in transporting personnel and equipment over the 90 miles from Port-au-Prince, the last 20 over a seemingly bottomless mud road.

In close association with the hospital, there was a community development program concerned with education and employment. Instruction and jobs were provided in woodworking, rug making, ceramics, sewing, pig and poultry raising. An elementary school, veterinary clinic, and a dairy herd and barn were close by. During my tenure a large modern chicken coop was the scene of a grand fete for all the staff to celebrate Dr.

Mellon's birthday the night before the chickens moved in.

A typical day began at 7 o'clock in the bright blue of a Haitian morning as I worked through the press of bodies crowding the entrance to the hospital sitting in the middle of that tortured island. I went immediately to x-ray where I sat with colleagues helping each other to read the problem films that had been culled from yesterday's cases, x-ray's we'd already read the evening before. One of us gets a "magnifique" for comparing a bunch of coiled ascaris in the abdomen with Van Gogh's "Starry Night," and another the gong for missing the calcification in a tuberculosis kidney. One of us three surgeons went to the O.R., the other made ward rounds.

I'd stay on the front steps deciding which of the 200 patients I'd admit and which ones I'd turn away, knowing full well that some had traveled as many as two days on foot. The clinics were already overflowing with people living in the hospital district who got total medical care, pills for worms or a pneumonectomy for a destroyed tuberculous lung, all for 40 cents. I sat the candidates on long benches in the shade so the sun wouldn't raise their skin temperature. I felt their pulse at the wrist. Was it rapid? Irregular? Thin from anemia or a wasting disease, or pounding from hypertension? I noted the skin temperature and pulled down the lower eyelid. Was the palpebral fissure white like my shirt, white in a woman who can still walk with chronic anemia and a hemoglobin of five? Was the conjunctiva suffused, the saffron hue of leptospirosis? Were there small nodules in the skin of the face and ears or was there the shiny silver spot of a new leprous infection on the arm? A goiter would be obvious, but I had to feel for tubercular cervical nodes and do another assessment of skin temperature. Was there a Casal's necklace of pellagra? Looking for tuberculosis or pneumonia, I asked for a cough and get a hint of congestive heart failure from the depth of the inhaling prior to the cough. I looked at the legs for the edema of congestive heart failure or tropical sprue. I lifted up shirts, checking for ascites. With women, I palpated through brightly colored dresses.

This screening took one minute: just sixty seconds to decide if the patient was in or out, perhaps to die if not admitted. In five of my nine years in Haiti, I personally screened, at nine in the morning and two in the afternoon, every Monday, Wednesday and Friday. Twice when I could no longer bear it, I got myself out of sight, had a good cry, then pulled myself together and went back to the benches. A pediatrician did the same for children. I was told not to fret too much because there were several other establishments where medical care was available.

I was curious about the options these people had for medical treatment, so I made a trip with Mimi and a driver in the hospital Land Rover, to visit each medical clinic from Port-au-Prince northward to determine where patients could get treatment for tuberculosis. We learned there were only two places north of Port-au-Prince besides us that were treating patients for tuberculosis. One was at Limbe with Dr. William Hodges and the other was the small Mennonite facility at Grand Riviere du Nord. Other places said they were doing fine and they did a lot of talking, but when I asked to see the pills, they turned out to be only vitamins, or there weren't any pills at all. They had been lying to me. That was particularly true of the major government hospital at Cape Haitian, an alleged tuberculosis hospital. Their "pills" proved to be solely vitamins, nothing else.

Tuesdays and Thursdays I was sequestered in the operating room doing what I did best and shielded from the administrative problems accruing to a medical director. On my way to the operating room, I usually passed Miss Pete's little cubbyhole office on the main corridor. She often beckoned me in and took my two hands between hers and said, "Bless these hands!" What a marvelous way to begin the day. Her full name was Walborg Petersen. Some years before, she and Betty Dumaine entered the nurses' training school at the Massachusetts General Hospital on the same day. Miss Pete was a "jick" from Brockton, Massachusetts. This colloquial term designated a recently arrived Englishman or woman working in the New England cotton mills. Miss Pete was not poor but of a low-income family, whereas Betty Dumaine was the daughter of Buck Dumaine who owned the New York, New Haven and Hartford Railroad and was a power in the upper strata of finance and society in New England. On that first day Ms. Dumaine debarked from a chauffeur-driven car with a fur coat and fancy luggage. Miss Pete walked in with a cheap straw suitcase. They became lifelong friends. When the Mellons asked Betty Dumaine some years later to suggest someone for superintendent of nurses, Betty suggested Miss Pete.

Miss Pete signed on early. She was a lovely, lovely woman. Sometimes I upset her, but one could never get mad at Miss Pete. Whether hot, dry or rainy, she always wore a crisp white uniform with her MGH cap and her MGH pin and a small embroidered white handkerchief in her upper left-hand pocket. Her white shoes were spotless. She did not wear stockings, but other than that she looked like a head nurse at the Massachusetts General. Indeed, she had been the assistant nursing supervisor of the Massachusetts Eye and Ear Infirmary before coming to Schweitzer. She, along with Larry and Gwen Mellon, made up the soul of the place.

The rest of the staff worked hard in the clinics and wards Monday through Friday, from seven in the morning to six or seven in the evening, with an hour for lunch. Saturday was a light half-day. All services were covered at night and on weekends by one of the ten physicians on rotation. All emergencies were handled first by the on-call physician for the whole hospital, and if he or she could not handle it, by an appropriate specialist. Ninety-five percent of those seeking help had significant organic disease. Each doctor had his own aide, read his own films, and did his own autopsies. There were no respirators and no fluoroscopes unless we had a visiting radiologist. Laboratory tests were carefully considered before ordering, the most common being a blood test for anemia, stools for parasites, smears for malaria and tuberculosis.

In this primitive area, peptic ulcer disease and cancer of the stomach were both common. The ulcer patients present with obstruction at the pylorus, the outlet of the stomach. In contrast, gall stones, appendicitis and colon cancer were rare. We took many chest x-rays but the only patient I ever saw with lung cancer was a heavy cigarette smoker from Port-au-Prince. We rarely saw arteriosclerosis in any form.

I never saw a patient with diverticulitis. Our experience was the same as that described by Dennis Burkett from Makerere University in Kampala, Uganda. He concluded that certain intestinal diseases are closely associated with diet. With adequate roughage, small and large bowel disease, including cancer, diverticulitis and appendicitis are rare. A British surgeon working for many years in Africa has said, "When I see an African with a bellyache who speaks English and has shillings in his pocket, he has appendicitis."

The average daily census was 160. Over half were pediatric cases and these were often bedded down two to three children to a crib. The hospital had no delivery service, but conducted an active prenatal clinic whose most important function was immunizing pregnant women with tetanus toxoid. In a woman never previously immunized, three shots of tetanus toxoid would prevent tetanus neonatorum in her infant for 5 to 10 years. We gave the first two shots a month apart, and the third in the last trimester. For a woman previously immunized, a booster shot in the last trimester is advised but not mandatory.

I was fifty years old, with much surgical experience behind me and the confidence and opportunity to tackle most anything surgical. And I did. My colleague, Dr. Harold May, and I were the only ones in the country who could open a chest or a head or turn out a good harelip and cleft palate. Harold was a long-time friend and chief of surgery at Hôpital Albert Schweitzer. As a surgeon I was under his authority, but as medical director I was over him.

We had a fine relationship. He was the son of a black Methodist minister and had inherited his father's missionary trait. Because of Harold's easy manner, integrity and sweetness of character, we never had major problems. His signal accomplishment was establishing an elementary school, one building and one grade at a time, progressing to about six grades. The school was a great success, but it began to erode into the care for his surgical patients. Harold suffered a blow when he was told to close the school. The details of the discussions and his leaving are murky, as Harold consumed his own smoke. He was a gentleman and did not confide in me or anyone else, although he did tell me that his offer to step down as chief of surgery and to work part time was refused. The public position of Dr. Mellon and Addison Vestal, Mellon's long-time friend and advisor, was that the charter of the hospital did not include schools.

A Yale relationship begun through the kindness of the chairman of surgery, Dr. Gustaf Lindskog, was the frosting on the cake. The men who were sent to us were at the end of their assistant residency, eager and brainy and pleasant. We had a wonderful time all learning together. Dr. May, a Yale resident, and I made up an unbeatable trio. I could sit there in the middle of that tragic island and be on the end of a pipeline that served me and the other full-time people the latest information brought by the Yale residents. The University of Cincinnati was already sending us pediatric residents, when I established a similar university connection with internists from the University of Vermont and pediatrics from Tufts. We developed a close association with the Harvard School of Public Health.

Dr. Marvin Sears, Chief of Ophthalmology at Yale, sent us residents year-round. Dr. Sears was introduced to us in this way. Once a month we had a compulsory journal club for the physicians. It was held on a late Tuesday afternoon after TB clinic had closed. Each chose an article from whatever journal he liked and reported on it. We stopped promptly at 5:30 p.m. I had chosen a 1967 article from *The Lancet* marking the twenty-fifth anniversary of the original 1942 landmark paper written by Sir Norman Gregg from Australia. Gregg had found that if a pregnant woman contracted German measles her baby might develop cataracts and other congenital deformities.

I was reporting on the paper when I received a call from the front desk announcing a doctor who wanted to see me. It was during the dry season and I went out to find a dusty white man, just off a camion, who identified himself as Dr. Marvin Sears, chairman of the Department of Ophthalmology at the Yale Medical School. He was touring around the Caribbean. Later he said he was looking for a place to send his residents to get additional training beyond the usual United States experience. He sat in with us, and he was taken off his feet when he saw that in this God-forsaken, desolate, and dusty Artibonite Valley in the middle of Haiti, there was a medical journal club with a surgeon, the medical director of the hospital, reporting on a seminal paper in ophthalmology. Thus began a continuing relationship with Dr. Sears's department, which sent many highly trained, personable young men to spend three to six months conducting a high-class ophthalmology service.

In an article for *The Rhode Island Medical Journal* I reported on a highly successful record of pulmonary surgery for tuberculosis. There were 500 cases, almost all resections with a 1.8 percent, 60-day mortality. Many things contributed to this. I was only two minutes away from the ward and if there were any immediate complications, I was there to remedy them. Also I put many patients preoperatively in the little tuberculosis lacour called "L'escale" where I made sure they had enough to eat and took their medicines. L'escale, a twelve-patient, bare-bones facility, was financed and built by Haitian doctors and staff as a halfway house for tuberculosis patients. It was made of cement blocks with windows high up so evil spirits could not spit on the patients as they slept. Some spent up to six weeks there until I thought they were in good condition and their x-rays had improved. Then I operated on them. Of all the pulmonary resections I did, perhaps 500 cases, I failed only on two as far as respiratory insufficiency was concerned. These patients lived, but they were confined to a chair and a few steps for their existence. At one time our test was the match test. We held a match within six inches of their mouth and if they could blow it out, they passed the test. After that we used something that had a balloon and a metal tube that worked by the venturi effect. Exonus was my helper in the clinic. He and I enveloped the patient, exhorting him to blow into the tube, coaching him, saying, "Respire' fo, pi fo, pi fo." for several minutes. The poor fellow would be all out of breath, but when he finished, and if he did pass, I did the resection. Most wanted the surgery because they knew they were going to be all right. One patient, who had not been ready for surgery by the time I left, threw himself in the Artibonite River.

Often during the pulmonary resections, none of my staff in the operating room had more than an eighth-grade education, including the anesthetist who had been trained by Dr. Garnier. There was Olga, the circulating person, who was not medically trained. She said little but was always there, and I was apprehensive when she was not. She knew just how to adjust the light and could handle all the demands put on a circulating nurse. Sometimes I wouldn't do a case unless Olga was there. Monny occasionally passed the instruments when the staff was short and assisted me with these pulmonary resection cases that could last four hours or longer. She would reluctantly assist at a child or infant hernia repair, reluctant because of the inadequacy she felt working with so few instruments instead of a big table filled with a multitude of tools.

It was a boon to us to train a young woman to become a capable auxilliare, skilled in a carefully defined task. And these new skills were a source of great pride to her. With the endorsement of Dr. and Mrs. Mellon and with the collaboration of my associate and best friend, Dr. Muller Garnier, we started a training school for nurses' aides. Dr. Rex Fendall of the Liverpool School of Tropical Public Health was our mentor. We trained young women from the local area who had only an eighth-grade education. We gave them a basic course for six months, and for the second six months trained them to do a specific task for which they would be particularly qualified. Therefore they became the experts, taking care of tetanus patients or helping me in the operating room or receiving special training in nutrition. This proved to be a great success for the patients, the hospital and for the auxiliaries themselves. It gave them jobs with us at the hospital, or elsewhere, furthering their confidence and self-esteem. "I am the scrub nurse for the Gros Chef Dr. Lepreau."

I developed several close friends at the hospital, but Muller Garnier was the dearest. He was committed to his country and to all things Hôpital Albert Schweitzer. He arrived early in my stay to learn anesthesia from our American Board certified Haitian anesthesiologist. Muller took over from him and in time trained several Haitian auxilliares to become qualified technicians. But Muller was much more than a good physician and anesthesiologist. He offered classes in French. When my 80-year-old mother came from Fall River to visit, he toured her around the countryside. He trained a mixed chorus that performed for Mme Mellon's birthday. At a lively party at our house, he quietly removed a Haitian who had become a bit enthusiastic. He became my associate and then followed me as medical director. When Monny and I were about to leave Haiti, Muller threw a magnificent dinner-dance-going-away party for us, complete with a 15-piece band, beans and rice and cabrite killed the same day.

Years later Muller developed metastatic lung cancer for which he received appropriate outpatient therapy at the Harlem Hospital in New York City. Monny and I visited him twice to check on his treatment and spirits. It was tragic to see the proud Muller Garnier holed up in two barren rooms below sidewalk level across from the Harlem Hospital. On our initial visit, when I asked to see his biopsy slides and x-rays, there was difficulty finding them. The Haitian underground had not registered him as a patient until his work-up had been completed, thanks to the New York City taxpayers. Old and new friends, alike, contributed funds for his care.

Upon my arrival at the hospital, I found a trio of outstanding Haitian internists, Francois Charles, Gerard Smarth and the prince, Rene St. Leger. St. Leger's expansive personality drew everyone to him. Tall, handsome, debonair and always first-class, he was a great party man. We clicked. St. Leger practiced alternately between East Illinois and Haiti, where he conducted a clinic for his poor countrymen to whom he remains devoted.

Another of my close friends in Haiti was Zeke Moura, a successful Lebanese businessman and a happy generous extrovert who did many favors for Monny and me. He had gone to two surgical shrines: the Mayo Clinic for a thyroid operation and to the Lahey Clinic for his gall bladder surgery. He came to me after I returned to Fall River for the removal of a chronically infected left submaxillary gland, which required delicate dissection but posed no threat to life. Dr. Robert Moe, a senior surgeon, assisted and Dr. Vincent Geremia was the anesthesiologist. They were two of the best. I was putting the dressing on when Zeke died, his pupils fixed. Everything was critically reviewed. The body was autopsied. I took the intact brain to Massachusetts General Hospital myself, where it was cut in my presence. No diagnosis. Perhaps hyperthermia. This was a profound tragedy for the extended Moura family and for me. With the deaths of Garnier and Moura and the separation from St. Leger, I lost a piece of myself.

In Haiti I learned there was more to the medical profession than surgery, particularly in public health. I hired the Berggrens, husband and wife physicians trained at the Harvard School of Public Health. Doctors Warren and Gretchen Berggren were a disparate couple.

They were both old-fashioned, evangelistic medical missionaries practicing in the Congo, just barely getting out before other American missionaries were assassinated. He was doing almost everything there, including surgery. Upon their return to the States they earned degrees from Harvard School of Public Health. We signed them on as our first public health people. Gretchen was a talker, but she had a good heart and a feel for Haitians. She did a lot for Harvard Public Health students who came to Haiti. Warren spoke little, but was very effective. They were in Haiti for five years and did a fantastic job.

For the first few months they looked at the hospital census and the entire hospital operation to decide what best to tackle, and picked tetanus because these patients filled many of the beds and required intensive nursing. Tetanus was easy to prevent by immunization which provided almost lifetime protection. Many infant cases resulted from the local custom of putting some unhygienic material on the umbilical cord stump. For a year and a half at dawn every Saturday morning, the tetanus immunization team gathered at the hospital. The team was led by a registered nurse, two petty officer types and some dollar-a-day lay people. They loaded their donkeys with equipment, left the hospital at 4:30 a.m. and headed to Petite Riviere, crossing the Artibonite on a makeshift wooden platform called a ferry, powered by an overhead pulley system to get the contraption across the river. On Saturdays people congregated at Petite Riviere for the market day. By late morning the team had immunized 4,000 people before returning in early afternoon. Dr. Warren Berggren went the first few times to get things organized, but subsequently a nurse was the only professional, keeping the cost at 33 cents for the three shots required per patient. It was a remarkable program and essentially wiped out tetanus in the valley. The experience in Haiti with tetanus has been written up and published in *The Lancet* (Feb. 15, 1975, pages 383-386) in a paper written by Muller Garnier, Florence Marshall, Kenneth Davison and me as well as in various other articles by Warren Berggren.

Simplify, simplify, simplify was our theme for treating those who did develop tetanus. Constant bedside care was the most important, and we provided it with a specially trained auxilliare working in a single room for four to six patients. The room was both noisy and bright. We had no respirators, and performed a rare tracheostomy accompanied by a gastrostomy. Diazepam was the exclusive sedative and relaxant. Wound care was standard with no antitoxin injected around the wound. Ten thousand units of tetanus antitoxin was about to be replaced with 500 units of human tetanus immunoglobulin. In a consecutive series of 985 cases from 1958 to 1972, the hospital mortality rate was 22 percent, possibly the best in the world for a large number of consecutive cases. There was considerable improvement in later years due to the simplified, dedicated bedside nursing and the use of only one sedative, the relaxant diazepam. For 1972, the last year of this study, we treated 72 newborn patients with a mortality of 25%.

The Berggrens were also involved in a nutrition outreach. In addition to the daily nutrition interview at the hospital, they inaugurated a nutrition center in surrounding villages educating mothers about choosing food from local markets that would improve their children's health and weight. Beans, of course, were the best, but often too expensive. Meat was not an option. Warren and Gretchen more than justified the faith we had in them to initiate a first class public health program. They were a huge success.

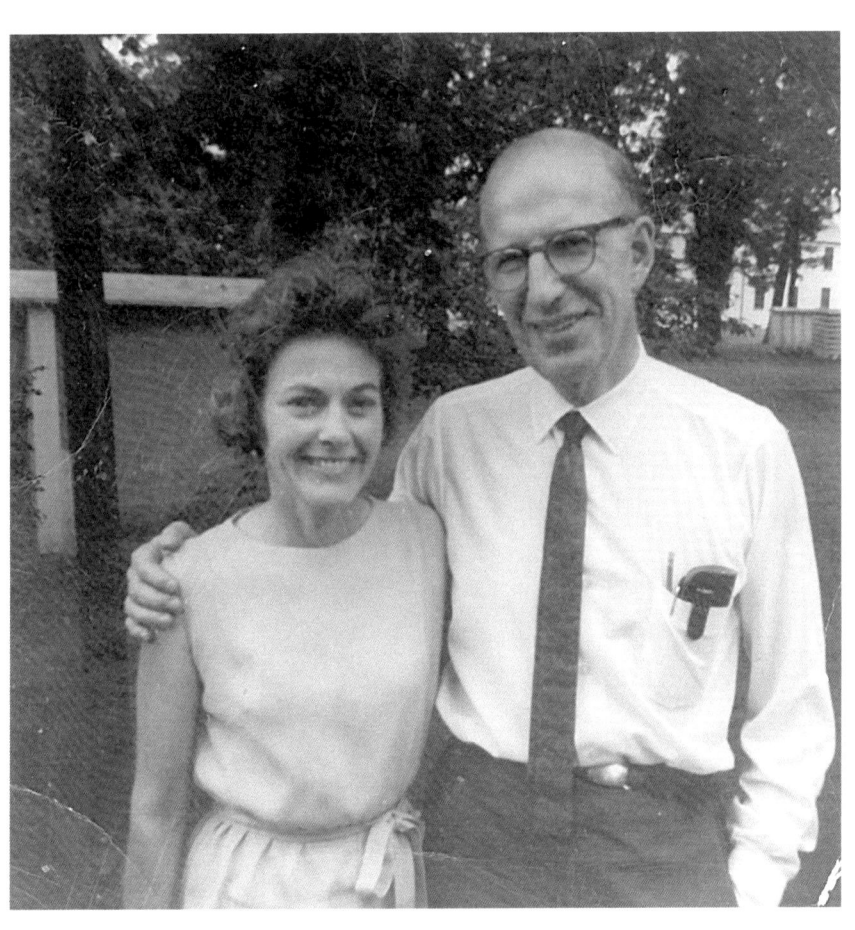

Monny and Frank - Haiti

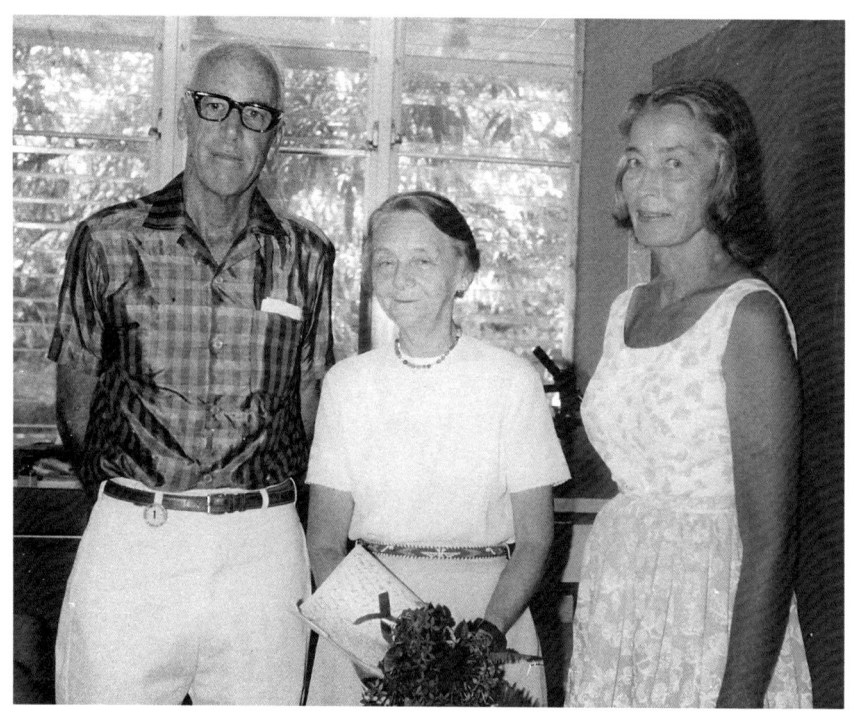

Keepers of the Flame
Dr. Larimer Mellon, Miss Pete and Gwen Mellon

9

Haiti — The Personal Side

Monny's contribution to the Haitian experience was boundless. Once there, she embraced the whole endeavor. One of the rich dividends of our Haitian experience was the closeness of our family, especially given the lack of compelling distractions beyond our home and the hospital compound. Monny and I and the children, Jay and Mimi, lived with no television, no trips to the movies, no automobile for our first few years. I did not find it a chore because I was so involved with the hospital. Monny was a self-starter, as usual, cooking, sewing and making the house pleasant. She occasionally went horseback riding. She home-schooled Jay and Mimi, which was not an easy task even with the aid of the Calvert correspondence system. She occasionally called me in for a parent-teacher conference. I cannot believe I was much help and probably muddied the waters.

The first year we were in Haiti we had a small cement block house with a common room, small kitchen, a bedroom for Monny and me and one for each child and a single bathroom. Later, we moved to a large stone house left over from the Standard Fruit Company days. Our new house had a wide screened-in expanse running the length of the house on the back. It was a perfect place to display our Paul Sample winter oil painting. It also made up for Monny's sacrifice in leaving behind her spacious country kitchen in Westport replete with all its appliances. Mrs. Mellon made a partial compensation by replacing a small outbuilding, formerly used as the kitchen, with an expansive new kitchen complete with an elaborate, newly purchased oven. Monny was happiest on Sundays when the servants were off and she had the kitchen to herself. But she was not alone. There in the new kitchen on a ledge above the sink lived Freddie, a small lizard, that with unerring accuracy would suddenly jump down and devour a cockroach. Monny and Freddie became good friends.

We enjoyed simple pleasures like the record player, card or board games. There was a Chinese game called "Go" at which Jay became reasonably proficient although I could never get the hang of it. We had hospital personnel to our house for supper and we went to their houses. With the Davisons and Garniers, we played a riotous card game called "In Between." We went to bed early. I always went to church on Sunday morning. Monny occasionally attended. Harold May was our ever-present pastor. After being up all Saturday night composing his sermon, he appeared fresh in a well-pressed white shirt resplendent against his black skin.

I tried to swim once a day. In the evening before going to bed I usually made a quick round on the surgical service and visited the other wards to see if there were any major problems. Altogether it was well-circumscribed, self-contained, simple life. The "work" day was long, hard and exhausting and I loved it. My relaxation was tennis on the weekends or in the evening after lights were installed on the court. It was not a hair shirt existence.

Monny reluctantly complied with the required three servants at $30 a month each. She and Carmen, a well-educated cook, worked with mutual respect. The houseman and laundress were a trial. Some years after we arrived, I, the medical director who was compulsive about employee health, found that Carmen had amoebiasis, the houseboy had hookworm and the laundress had never been immunized for tetanus. Most of the time our family was healthy, but Monny contracted a moderately severe case of dengue, Mimi became seriously ill with measles, Jay contracted hepatitis with jaundice, and my productive cough became worse. The cough was due to an allergy to rats, which ran around over our beaverboard ceiling. One time Monny opened our clothes closet and there was one on a shelf staring her down.

At the hospital Monny coded all the in- and out-patient diagnoses, which was a great help to the Berggrens, in their goal to establish a hospital census track of 10,000 people. For pleasure, Monny rode our horse, Shelley, and occasionally rode to Verrette five miles away for supplies. One day I remember her returning from there over a muddy road in a downpour while carrying a bolt of cloth under her poncho. She could do anything, and was totally supportive of all of us.

One of the tasks I assigned to Jay when he was young was to determine why the milk was contaminated. It was a classic public health project and he came up with the right answer. I instructed him to watch the milk from the time it left the cow until it finished processing. He found a break in technique that occurred when the attendant in the milk house poured the milk out of a bucket whose rim had been in the milk handler's hand just minutes before. Doctor Boltax, a Yale assistant in surgery, had grown up in Columbia where his father had a big farm, and he participated in this venture.

Tennis was a big part of our social activity. I considered myself to be an ordinary player but some of the visitors and Jay were good. I recall a remarkable doubles match between Dr. Robert Bellows, an ophthalmologist resident from New Haven, Dr. Steve Stein, a Yale surgical resident and Dr. Marvin Sears. I don't recall the fourth person, but it may have been Jay or Ken Davison. The tennis court was an ancient cement court with several cracks in it, but it still worked. Playing during daylight could be hot and uncomfortable, so we besought Dr. Mellon to put in lights, allowing us to play at night. This was a great concession on his part, and we all enjoyed it. I remember playing doubles with the well-known Haitian art critic, Selden Rodman, and his current wife as well as his ex-wife.

The Mellons had guests of all stripes. One time when Monny was with Sue and her newborn in Georgia, Mrs. Mellon asked Mimi to host a luncheon for some female friends from the States. I think they included one or two of Larry's sisters, a Havemyer and maybe a Rockefeller. Mimi, in her early teens, was just right — pleasant, respectful, not intimidated, and carried the conversation without monopolizing it.

The only family negative of our overseas experience was our isolation from good secondary education. When Jay and Mimi reached high school age we had to make a decision. Should they attend the Union School, an American private high school in Port-au-Prince, or go to the States to stay with close friends or relatives and attend local schools or attend a boarding school? We finally decided on Westtown, an excellent Quaker school near West Chester, Pennsylvania. This was a good choice. I think Monny's friend, Kenney Rea, paid the tuition for one year or more for Mimi. We made sure that we could finance the trip home for every vacation. We remained a close foursome in spite of the time the children spent away from home during their high school years.

Jay went off first and had a difficult time. He was lonesome, which resulted in a tense few days for all of us at the end of his first Christmas vacation. Monny took Jay to Port-au-Prince to put him on the plane. She left him at the Oloffson Hotel while she went downtown to shop. When she returned Jay was missing. Monny panicked. Where was this teenager in a large tropical city? There was a lot of unsuccessful quasi-official activity searching for a young white boy. I came home from the hospital about six o'clock and found Jay sitting on his bed. I did not know how to react. I was furious, but I held my tongue. Jay just didn't want to go back to school. He was fluent in Creole and had hopped a camion and came home. Mr. DeVastey took me to Verrettes where an ancient telephone allowed us to get word to the Oloffson telling Monny that Jay was home.

We finally persuaded him to return for the second semester of his first year. We made a deal with him that he reluctantly accepted. The following year Mimi would be going to Westtown. If, after spending the first semester of his second year with Mimi, he still was unhappy, he could come home. As we were putting him in the Land Rover in the custody of an old friend, Dr. James Hennessey, I looked him in the eye and he looked me in the eye. I will never forget the poignant words we exchanged. I said, "Jay, is there anything I can do for you?" He responded, "Yes, Dad. Don't send me back." That was heart-rending.

He continued at Westtown doing well. He was a good runner and I watched him compete. He was captain of the track and cross-country team. He got the top ranking scholarship in the school, meaning he had one year of tuition at Haverford College. We were all very proud of him. At Haverford Jay became addicted to all things computer and after a year and a half spent in the computer center, he was invited out of there and out of the college.

During Jay's time at home, both before and after Westtown and Haverford, we had a good time together. He helped me and assisted as a translator in the clinic. I was fair at Creole but not nearly as competent as Jay. He scrubbed with me in the O.R. particularly on difficult vesico-vaginal fistulas, which I had taught myself from books. He had many Haitian friends of all ages and they loved to banter with him, a typical Haitian diversion. A few of Jay's Haitian friends occasionally precipitated a problem with Carmen, our cook, because the Haitian friends were of a lower social class and Carmen wasn't pleased to wait on them at the table.

Jay had a horse, which provided some adventures. One occurred during the dry season when there was no green grass for the horse. The only continuing good source nearby was Madame Mellon's yard, and that caused me problems. In my official state I had to side with her. As a parent I did not want to hound Jay, so I just left things alone. But it was a "cops and robbers" event between Mrs. Mellon and her watchmen chasing Jay off the fields and Jay avoiding them by moving the horse at night. I learned much later that she was furious.

After Jay came back from Haverford, he was mixed up and worked in the laboratory as a salaried employee. Then he became an assistant to two good American internists and actually could run the clinic pretty much himself. So I asked Dr. Mellon if Jay could take over and run one of the medical clinics, with or without pay, when one of the long-termers left in a couple of weeks. His answer was no. Jay could stay on at the lab for the standard $150.00 a month, but that was all. Dr. Mellon's decision was a disappointment. It seemed to be a critical time in Jay's life. It was the end of 1972 and staying in Haiti, working in the medical clinic, like a nurse practitioner or an intern, would have been a considerable help to Jay at a crucial time in his life.

Soon after we arrived in Haiti we became acquainted with Sister Joan Margaret, an Anglican nun and the only person in Haiti who was trained in and did anything in physical therapy. Sister Joan was a saint: short, a bit round and usually wearing a beautiful smile. We had a close association with her and she gave Mimi, at the age of twelve, a job as the waterfront instructor and monitor for her camp in Montrouis. I think it was Mimi's first extended experience away from home and everyone had a good time. It was kind of Sister Joan to put this much faith in Mimi, but she was a smart woman and knew what she was doing.

I clearly remember the first time I met Sister Joan. I was on a plane headed back to the States sitting in a seat near the front. A nun with flowing black robes stepped on with a bundle under one arm and a typewriter on the other. The bundle turned out to be a young Haitian boy named Oneikel who had neither arms or legs. I timidly engaged her in conversation at sometime during the flight. She said she was bringing Oneikel up to a place in northern New Jersey to be fitted for prostheses.

There were three doctors from Atlanta--Jim Funk, Robert Wells and Skoot Dimon--who took turns doing elective orthopedic surgery for us three times a year. Most of the patients were those that Sister Joan had rounded up during the previous four months. We did the surgery and then sent them back to her for rehabilitation. She drove a huge Toyota Land Rover loaded up with her patients, bringing them in for orthopedic week and then taking them back to her place for physio or returning them to their homes, mostly on the south coast. One time Monny and I went with her when she was delivering some of these children home, and the Land Rover was crowded. As we were loading up, she said in a loud voice, "Oneikel, take off your arms and legs and have somebody put them on the roof." And that is exactly what happened.

We had many contacts with Sister Joan, all of them marvelous. On her desk, in the middle of her tumultuous clinic, she had a small picture of a sailboat with a sign beneath it saying, "It isn't how hard the wind blows, it is how the sails are set." Sister Joan was one of those we stopped to say goodbye to as we were leaving the country. At the convent gate I said, "Sister Joan, you have meant so much to our family and to me professionally and yet we have not seen all that much of you. Now we are leaving today." She replied, "Friendship does not depend on the frequency of contact, it is just knowing that the other person is there."

~

Mimi made out very well in Haiti. She could adapt to almost anything. She became fluent in the language. She fraternized with the maids and cooks and must have known all the gossip about the place, none of which came back home. Actually there was not much gossip there that amounted to anything. We all got along well. One interesting sidelight on the news was the beagle, Bulldozer, that we brought from the States and gave to the Mellons. After becoming oriented, Bulldozer, in typical beagle fashion, made early morning rounds of all the residents hoping for a snack. We joked that he must have been fitted with a tape recorder so he could return with a report to Madame Mellon who liked to know what was going on.

Mimi spent much of her time with the various veterinarians, becoming knowledgeable and of considerable help to them. When she was departing for Westtown, I told her that she was going to meet a lot of sophisticated young women. I encouraged her not to be daunted by them. She said, "Don't worry about me, Daddy. I bet none of those girls know how to do a pregnancy test on a cow." A pregnancy test on a cow means putting on a rubber gauntlet up to the armpit and putting one's hand and arm into the rectum to determine if the uterine arteries are pulsating. If they are pulsating, the animal is pregnant.

Another time when there seemed to be considerable violence in the United States, she was on her way back to school. She carried an open basket on her arm and protruding from it was a heavy nickel-plated steel instrument for castrating pigs. When I said something about taking care of herself, she said, "Don't worry about me, Daddy. I'll take care of those guys."

At parties Mimi was a great success. She danced the merengue well and occasionally made parodies on Tom Lehrer songs and played them on the piano. I recall seeing her in the middle of our living room when we were having a dance. She said, "Come dance with me." She worked many hours on those long hot days in the clinic, especially when Skeets was running them so late, sometimes until ten or eleven at night.

As I think about the children, I think our time in Haiti was a great experience for them as it was for the whole family. Monny and I made out well. One time, perhaps on an anniversary, we went "out on the town." We had a large living room with a cement floor. We got all dressed up. I might have put on my tuxedo. Monny was all gussied up in a lovely long dress. We went to one corner of the room for cocktails and then to another corner for an appetizer. Working our way around our own living room, we had our main meal and finally coffee and dancing.

Occasionally when I was able to get away for a weekend we went to Port-au-Prince on the hospital bus, and later, in our own car, after five years without one. We spent our time at the Oloffson Hotel, which was absolute relaxed luxury. We tried to book Chambre B where I had taken Monny when she first came to Haiti. It had a balcony covered with bougainvillea overlooking the pool.

The Oloffson had been a United States Marine Hospital during their 1914 to 1933 occupation. When we were in Haiti, it had become a rambling wooden structure presided over by an unusual couple, Sue and Al Seitz. Sue Seitz had come to the Caribbean with a close female friend touring on a shoestring for the fun of it. They came out to our hospital one October looking for jobs. We signed them up to return in January and, *mirabile dictu*, they did. Sue, who was not too physically active but had a lot of brains, was put in the record room. She did a great job. They lived in one of the smaller cement houses and used to have some wild parties, especially on weekends. They made a lot of noise which Gwen didn't like, but Sue did her job so well that Madame Mellon could do nothing about it. Sue eventually married Al Seitz, and they became a perfect match to run and maintain the legendary hospitality of this kooky hostelry.

The Oloffson usually hosted a dance on Saturday night and occasionally a voodoo show. Several American and foreign celebrities stayed at this quirky place. On one of my visits, a well-known television newsman became seriously ill. I helped take care of him, but he was near death. Mrs. David Brinkley was there at a dance. It was a collection of artists, writers and journalists including the ever-present Haitian journalist, Aubelin Jolicouer.

Jolicouer was a small, slender dandy who seemed to know everything but told you nothing. He always carried a walking stick about three feet long. He once left it on a low table while he and I were having a drink together and it rolled off. I picked it up, noting of how heavy it was, probably solid iron. He was an enigmatic figure. He helped Monny, the children, and me once or twice when we were having trouble with customs. But, although he seemed to take a liking to us, I remained wary.

Twice during our time in Haiti, one of the big bands like Nemours John-Baptiste came out with twelve musicians, gratis, to liven up the atmosphere. Wet or dry, it was a miserable hot trip from Port-au-Prince and back. They used our house to clean up. They were soaking wet and full of mud in the wet season, and they were covered with dust in the dry season. They began playing at eight o'clock and finished around one in the morning with one twenty-minute break. Their only compensation was food and rum. It was a blast and a tremendous contribution to the hospital community. The second time they performed for a party at the clubhouse on Halloween. Everyone was in costume, most noteworthy being the short Mike Curci on stilts and dressed as a woman. Many of us did not know who he was for a long time. Skeets was dressed as a Haitian peasant in a typical blue denim dress from Ternette.

One evening we were returning from Port-au-Prince in our Volkswagen station wagon when the lights picked up a well-dressed couple crossing a stream with a donkey. The woman had dismounted and was bare-legged, seeking the shallowest place to cross. In contrast the husband remained astride the donkey with legs pulled high to keep them dry. I said "Well, Monny?" But she had not become that Haitian. She stayed put and we followed the Madame safely across.

I spent considerable time with the Mennonites on my first two trips to Haiti when I was there on my own. They befriended me, and I went on many of their simple excursions. They were a great group mostly from the central United States, Pennsylvania, and Canada, and came from farm backgrounds. The men seemed able to do anything; when Dr. Mellon had a big project, he gave it to the Mennonites. He would outline it for them; they asked a couple of questions and then disappeared. When they reappeared a few days or weeks later, the project would be complete.

On my first trip I was green, apprehensive and scared. One evening, one of the Mennonites, Maggie Schrock, who was helping me in the clinic said, "Do you want to go down to the sugar mill?" I agreed and off I went following the small young woman in her flip-flops with her blonde ponytail bobbing up and down in front of me. On a twisting path through the inky blackness we passed tree trunks that seemed like voodoo spirits ready to pounce.

We arrived at the sugar mill, which was operating at night to avoid the heat of the sun. In the center of a clearing were three upright wooden cylinders about three feet high and a foot in diameter, two of them abutting the central one. The power source was a twelve-year-old boy at the end of a fifteen-foot-long horizontal bar. The boy walked around and around at the end of the bar, which was connected to the central cylinder which, in turn, engaged the other two. Men or boys then advanced two or three stalks of sugar cane between the cylinders which squeezed the juice which ran off into a receptacle. When the container was full, the juice was taken to a cauldron to boil down over a hot wood fire producing something that looked like molasses. Occasionally, at the hospital, a boy would be brought in with a severe crushing injury of his hand or arm. He had become sleepy and had forgotten to take his hand off the sugar cane.

After Monny and I became long-term residents, I still maintained the relationship with the Mennonites. Monny did also. She taught the young wives how to cook and sew. Many of them had come from farms so they already knew the technique, but not the art. There was a strict rule that these young men and women in their late teens and twenties, could not have any love affairs. One time, however, two of them, Charlie Harms and Margaret Smith, fell in love, and it prompted me to write:

> There was a young woman named Smithy
> Who found her lover far away from the city.
> Now in Kansas he plows
> While in Haiti she bows
> To the whims of the Central Committee.

And that is what happened. I occasionally attended a Mennonite bible study. At one of the sessions, the current veterinarian, who was a Catholic, went with me. The group had a long discussion about the meaning of various words and phrases in the Bible. Finally my veterinary friend said, "Hey, folks, you know we Catholics and our monks had that book in the back room of our monasteries for decades, or maybe centuries, and we modified it just the way we wanted it."

~

It was in 1969 while I was in Haiti that I had the opportunity to spend some time at the Grenfell Mission in northern Newfoundland. I had visited the Grenfell office in Boston in 1947 to inquire about a position there as chief of surgery. I knew that Dr. Curtis, who had followed Dr. Grenfell, was looking for a successor.

However, Dr. Gordon Thomas, a much better qualified man than I, took the position. He was a Canadian and an outdoor man well acquainted with the sea and the North. The Grenfell Mission in northern Newfoundland and Labrador was founded in 1900 by Dr. Wilfred Grenfell, a true medical missionary. The Grenfell was well-known to those growing up in my generation as the place to go for adventure, medical care, and other do-good experiences. Tuberculosis, vitamin deficiency and malnutrition were common. Years later in 1969, I met Dr. Thomas at a tuberculosis meeting in the Dominican Republic. We were on the same wavelength. He came and spent a week with me at Hôpital Albert Schweitzer, then stayed at Schweitzer for a month while I went to St. Anthony and took over for him.

We shared the same attitudes towards life and surgery, so the exchange was pleasant and we both enjoyed it. I went on my way to Deer Lake in a commercial plane and was met there by the mission plane. I expected someone like Jack London to get out of the plane all done up in winter flying garb. The pilot who emerged from the plane was wearing a fedora hat, a long black New York City type overcoat, and black oxfords.

On the coast, I wanted to see or ride in a dogsled, but the only dog I saw was running alongside my skidoo, a one passenger motorized sled. All along the jagged coast and into Labrador, there were nursing stations occupied by two nurses who took care of the medical needs of all the people. The communities were often found at the bottom of the cliffs on the shores of small bays. The nurses were rugged types from the old days. When they were driving a dog team they always carried a revolver because the dogs could get out of hand. Jay and Mimi accompanied me. We had a nice apartment, but Mimi went into a cocoon and promptly left. Lucy Ann joined us later and then returned again as the Grenfell's first social worker.

Lucy had been on her way to Grenfell Mission a few years before to spend a summer at St. Anthony, but fate dealt her a cruel blow. She had a benign acoustic neuroma. Dr. Donald Matson, one of the best surgeons in the world, removed the tumor at the Peter Bent Brigham Hospital. The operation left her with a unilateral facial paralysis, a complication that was expected in acoustic neuroma surgery at the time. Now the tumor is usually excised through the auditory canal with no facial nerve injury. Matson died prematurely of a mysterious degenerative condition later known as Jakob-Creutzfeldt disease, a slow virus similar to Kuru, made known to the world by the extraordinary field work in New Guinea by another Harvard Medical School graduate, Carleton Gajdusek. Matson's autopsy tissue was retrieved to confirm the diagnosis.

At St. Anthony I did quite a bit of surgery with satisfactory results. The equipment and operating room staffs were fine. I did several gallbladder operations, the condition probably due to obesity and the high fat diet. The food was adequate but high in fat. A popular meal was called Fishermen's brewis: white potatoes and white fish swimming in bacon grease, served on a white plate.

I visited L'anse aux Meadows on the extreme northern tip of Newfoundland, the site of the only proven permanent Viking settlement in the Americas, active around 900 A.D. The critical artifact was a stone disk, 5 to 6 inches in diameter, with a hole in the center, part of a spinning apparatus used by women of Norway at the time. It was found by Tony Beardsley, son of Hartness Beardsley, one of my close friends in college. The young Beardsley was about sixteen and was a pick and shovel excavator on the well-established dig. At the close of the season he said to the people in charge, "May I do a little digging on my own?" He was granted permission but told to stay outside the perimeter. So he began digging and found the disk that was the key to the timing and authenticity of the permanence of the Viking settlement at L'anse aux Meadows, the first one in the New World.

Dr. Gordon Thomas was an old hand in the hard north in the early days of the Grenfell, mushing with dog teams, breaking through ice in a boat and then flying. He took Lucy Ann and Jay and me over the northern part of the island in his plane. The coastline is jagged and knife-edged with innumerable coves and bays that are narrow, often with no connection to the main part of the island without scaling a cliff. I recall that James Cook's detailed mapping of the Newfoundland coast was so well done that the admiralty took notice of him. Thereafter his career was meteoric.

On our return trip Lucy Ann, Jay and I stopped at Harty and Peg Beardsley's home at Deer Lake in the middle of Newfoundland. Harty was a contemporary from Dartmouth and a good friend. He and Peg had been in Newfoundland for years. He was the manager of the local Bowater hydropower plant, made up of eight low maintenance turbines that had been running since 1900. Isolated as Peg was up there in the frozen north, the small greenhouse room attached to their house led her to an interest in weather. She set up a telescope and became a significant part of the North American weather monitoring system. It doesn't matter where you are. If you have the ambition you can get a job anywhere.

~

One of my colleagues in Haiti was Florence Nightingale Marshall, better known as Skeets or Dr. Marshall in the Deschapelles community. Skeets was a trip, but a wonderful, crusty, loving friend and a pediatrician devoted to her sick children. "You can change anything else around here but don't interfere with my children." Hôpital Albert Schweitzer opened in 1956 and Skeets began the first of many six- to eighteen-month tours in the fall of 1957 continuing through 1980.

Our children adored Skeets, and she and Monny were good friends. On weekends after the early afternoon nap, we played tennis on the hot, cracked, cement court and then shared a couple of glasses of Heineken. She was a great party person, often showing up in the dark blue denim dress worn by the ladies from Ternette. At a birthday party for Larry Mellon, she sang "Don't Fence Me In" accompanied by guitar. In 1998 she was working three days a week in the Pediatric AIDS clinic at the New York Hospital.

An interesting episode evolved with Skeets. She was running her pediatric clinics up to eleven o'clock at night with the heat and the humidity getting worse and worse. Both she and the supporting staff, laboratory and x-ray personnel were becoming saturated with the heavy workload. It became too much. Skeets let herself get out of hand and I didn't seem able to control the situation. Dr. Mellon approached me one time and said, "Frank, you must get her to cut those clinics down." Telling someone like Skeets Marshall, who was devoted to patient care and especially to sick children, to stop caring for them was worse than trying to break down the Berlin wall. No way! I tried various approaches without success.

Since we were both Quakers, I thought I would try the Quaker approach. I figured out a reasonable quid pro quo and one day I said, "Hey, Skeets, may I come over and see you tonight after supper?" She agreed and later I went over to her small cement block house. It turned out that she sat in one corner and I sat in the opposite corner just like a couple of boxers. In less than five minutes I had presented my program. I decided to wait her out so I sat for thirty minutes in my corner. She sat for thirty minutes in her corner. I got up and said "See ya," She got up and said "See ya". I left and nothing more passed between us.

Some ten days later the clinics slowly, ever so slowly, began to get smaller and smaller. A few weeks later a call came from the front steps: "Dr. Marshall wants to see you." I went and there she was in a crowd of hot, sweaty mothers and children. Skeets had a typical dehydrated marasmic child with peeling skin draped over her extended arms. "OK, Frank, Goddamit, what do you want me to do with this?"

Dr. Chad Squires, a young graduate, well-trained in internal medicine, joined our staff and his wife, Joan, took over the running of the laboratory. While Squires was with us, Joan became pregnant. She was about thirty-three years old, and this was her first pregnancy. We had a good English midwife and Joan wanted to be delivered at our hospital. Everybody knew that, although I was the senior doctor and knew a fair amount, I was not qualified to handle serious obstetrical problems. However, being the senior person, I was ultimately responsible.

Joan went into labor under the care of our midwife and had a long hard labor, constantly observed and coached by the midwife. The fetal heart remained good and no meconium showed. I was in and out of the small minor operating room. There were two young pediatricians in training from New York Hospital with us, and they were so antsy about the fetus that they urged me to do something, badgering me every time I came out of the room. I wasn't too sure myself, but it got to me after a while. It made me wonder whether I was doing the right thing by sitting it out. Finally I couldn't stand the heat any longer. I locked myself in the small room with the midwife and Joan and didn't go out again, afraid to be put on the rack by these young tyros. Joan delivered a nice big healthy baby whom these pediatricians thought would be maimed for life. The baby went on to become valedictorian of her high school in New Hampshire and subsequently graduated from Swarthmore.

During Chad's tenure, Dr. Mellon had several episodes of a mixture of auricular fibrillation and auricular flutter, which is a serious irregularity of the heart. He had been treated by other physicians passing through and by cardiologists of some repute in Port-au-Prince. Most of the time he was asymptomatic but occasionally it got the best of him. During one of these cardiac episodes, Mrs. Mellon ordered Squires and me to come down to talk over Dr. Mellon's cardiac situation. Rightly so, she was concerned about her husband and grilled Squires severely. He held up pretty well considering he was young in the profession and apt to be intimidated by the Madame's authority and knowledge.

It was during one of these episodes that my colleague, Dr. Harold May, contacted a close friend at the Massachusetts General Hospital, who was a skilled cardiologist. We talked him into coming down to shock Dr. Mellon, that is, put an electrical charge through his heart to return the rhythm to normal. He came with several boxes of equipment, which in those days was much more cumbersome than now. As he had to return promptly to Boston, we did the procedure the evening he arrived.

The event was dramatic. We could see the black of night through the small high operating room windows. Darkness prevailed inside as well where the only light was the powerful overhead operating room light shining down on Dr. Mellon as he lay on the table waiting for the current to be turned on. We were a skeleton crew with each person assigned to one task. Dr. Garnier gave a light anesthesia. The visiting doctor stood in the midst of a pile of electrical equipment. As he put the plate on Dr. Mellon's sternum and threw the switch, Dr. Mellon sat three-quarters up and then lay back, his arms outstretched to the side. Good Night! This looked like a disaster. Had we killed him? Of course not. His rhythm returned to normal.

Addison Vestal was the financial guru for Larry Mellon going way back to his early manhood. We physicians wanted to open beds on Ward 3, which was really a store room with a couple of apartments on one end. This was a financial problem. Addison wouldn't let us do it, so I turned out the following verse.

I'm Addison Vestal from Pitt.
The income and outcome don't fit.
You will have to eat rice,
I can't pay the price,
And Ward 3 you will have to forgit.

At one of the annual meetings I was sitting with Everett Radovsky, as Addison went on and on about the past history of his relationship with Larry Mellon and the hospital. It was deadly. Dr. Everett Radovsky whispered to me, "Well, there is one thing worse than a bore and that is a bore with total recall."

Because of my official position, we had many dinner guests. There was always a steady stream of short-term staff and occasionally a large group of old friends like Skeets Marshall, Ken and Maureen Davison and Dr. Chad Squires and his wife Joan. We were pleased to have the newcomers to dinner because they brought news from old friends and places, and brought us up to date on what was happening at Yale and elsewhere. At one of our parties I dressed up in an operating room gown and made a big to-do with the Mennonites who wanted their ears pierced. Monny worked along with Carmen, our cook, to prepare for these dinners. Carmen would do the shopping in Petite Riviere or St. Marc, returning with a basket of produce on her head. Monny would do the planning and much of the cooking and Carmen would be there for the cleaning up. It was fun, but we soon learned that tomorrow was another hot, busy day beginning at 7 a.m. and not to end until twelve hours later. We decided that for the Mellons and the

Lepreaus the standard going home time would be 9:30 p.m.

Dr. Mellon felt he should do his part in running the hospital and participating in its activities. Once he conducted a church service, which was difficult for him. He didn't like to talk about himself or things sentimental but he did it, reading about love from a small book which had belonged to his mother. He was dripping with perspiration and his blue shirt was soaking wet when he finished. This is the only time I saw him preside at church. At other hospital social functions, he joined in by playing his guitar and concertina.

Before leaving Haiti in 1973, I wanted to follow up the tuberculosis patients on whom I had performed lung resections. Many of them lived in the mountains of distant Perodin. Devika Frankenbach was willing to help. Devika was an exceptionally able, attractive and energetic nurse who came to us after five years at Lambarene, where her first six months were spent working in the vegetable gardens. When asked how she liked it she replied, "Fine, except when I had diarrhea and had to run thirty meters in a tropical downpour to the outhouse."

Devika and I made the trip in March, the hottest time in the Artibonite. The summer heat had begun but not the cooling summer showers. Devika and two horses, each loaded with huge baskets called makouts, arrived on our front steps at 4 a.m. Off we went across the wide Artibonite valley and then up, up all day in the broiling sun. Lunch was in the "shade" of a small bush. This was followed by a long trek of more than a mile, much of it wading and pulling the horses through a shallow ten-foot wide streambed. Half way up, an underground river emptied into our stream from beneath a fifty-foot bank, which had an opening fifteen feet wide by ten feet high with the water four feet deep. We stripped to our underwear and went in exploring amongst the tangled roots, birds, and insects on either side and in the roof. We went in about two hundred feet, after which it became too dark and scary. I felt like Tom Sawyer with Becky Thatcher looking for Injun Joe.

We turned back to the horses to dry and change and then started up the streambed which became narrower, steeper and deeper. The water rushed more swiftly making it difficult to remain on our feet. At one point I pulled my packhorse up the stream and stumbled upon a lonely cemetery about fifty years old, with its markers rotting away. We were far out in the country. Water and greenery were being replaced by rock. It had been a long haul and I was beat out despite the fact that I had trained by running up the hill by our house for the past three weeks.

As the day wore on, we grew increasingly hot and tired in the relentless sun. My horse was skinny and so tired and beaten up he couldn't handle it. He fell into a crevice in the solid rock. We could barely get him out and away. Then, in the late afternoon, with the sun still beating down on the rocky landscape, we came across two postulants in full habit sitting on the trail with thermos bottles of hot coffee. They had been sent out by the priest to nourish and guide us in. That evening the priest prepared a fabulous meal, opening a large tin containing a whole Danish ham. I was embarrassed that he had gone to such an effort for us. He should have saved it for himself. I slept upstairs on the bare floor and slept well because I was so tired.

The next day was misty and wet, almost raining. We went to Mass given by our host where we met several of our old tuberculosis patients. After Mass the priest took his walking stick and, wearing rubber boots, strode down the hill on a muddy trail and disappeared into the fog on his way to another service four miles away. It reminded me of Stevenson's *Travels with a Donkey*.

The next evening we stayed at a small residence with nuns and the postulants. The young women put on a show for us on the front porch. It was a comedy accompanied by much singing. I was not allowed to sleep in the same building with the nuns and Devika. They put me in the chapel on a pallet in a small space behind the altar, a statue of Jesus looking down on me to keep me straight. It was a beautiful moonlit night with the air just the right temperature. Close by the chapel, a meandering stream, shallow and clear with extensive beds of watercress, ran through the field. I was transported by the romance of it and sat down to write a long letter to Max Eddy in Vermont who had helped us at the Hôpital. I wrote it by light of a candle, maybe two candles. I'm sure I was carried away.

We returned via a long, hot descent across open rocky slopes. Devika amazed me by saying she would soon prepare refreshments in the "shade" of a tree trunk far away at the bottom of the hill. Once there, she produced bread and rolls, cheese, water, charcoal and kerosene from her pack. The food and hot tea were refreshing.

For Monny and me it was a major project to ride around the countryside on the bad roads, carrying extra wheels and supplies in our vehicle, and we did little of it. We once went to Saut d'eau with Lucy Ann and Stuart

Polk. The waterfall nearby was a hundred feet high and was the center of voodoo worship in our part of Haiti. Thousands of people were swarming there for the annual renewal of their faith on July 15th. Another time we went south with Sister Joan to Cayes and to Isle la Vache, a small island off the coast where we all went swimming, even Sister Joan in her habit. I have a picture of her soaking wet within all those dripping folds.

Shortly before we left Haiti, Monny and I made a trip to visit Father John Breslin at Mole St. Nicholas, an ancient, crumbling French fort guarding the entrance to Mole's large, deep harbor, once considered an alternate to Guantanamo. We saw a small stream, controlled by the local commandant, trickling into the gardens, mostly his own. Young men were playing guitars made from five-gallon oilcans and fish line. It was a barren isolated landscape. We walked on a moonlit beach with soft curling white surf and saw an abandoned white stone seminary building, bright in the moonlight. In the harbor were three American motorized pleasure boats and a Haitian sailboat on its way to Port-Au-Prince loaded with charcoal for cooking and heating, perhaps the last phase in the destruction of that island. It began long ago when treeless Spain needed wood to build its Navy. Ah, war. It reaches everywhere and has no half-life. The avenger of our time will be nuclear waste, "the sins of the fathers."

At Father Breslin's medical clinic I was up at 6:00 a.m. sitting on the edge of an old army cot. At the other end was a lady about to give birth to her fourth baby. Father Breslin had been up with her since 1:00 a.m. Emma, a nurse's aide, had been with her all night. The lady simply bore down in silence. There were two big wash pans on the floor and a sink with running water, supplied from an elevated cistern filled by a three-bladed water-pumping windmill built by Father Breslin. At the other end of the cot was a box of powdered milk. Another lady had her baby about 6:30 a.m. and went home by 8:00 a.m. John Breslin gave no tetanus toxoid for immunizations because he was afraid he would be accused of taking over for the Sante Publique. Tetanus immunization prevents a common Haitian malady, tetanus of the newborn, which can be 90 percent fatal. Later I performed several surgical procedures under local anesthesia, which I had learned during residency days by studying Labat's classical text on the subject.

I subsequently developed a major pain in a finger of my right hand. I was convinced that it was an acute infectious tenosynovitis. I was frightened for there were no potent antibiotics there and I felt it necessary to leave Mole at once. By complete chance, the Haitian president's helicopter landed with United States or Canadian businessmen who were surveying the area for a possible resort. I packed up all our things, took our bags over to the helicopter and pled my case with the commander. Could he somehow provide a ride for Monny and me? We waited. In half an hour the plane was ready to go and he motioned for us to get in for the trip back to Port-au-Prince. The helicopter flew low with the doors open. Despite the emergency of my condition and the fear we had of falling out, we enjoyed the excitement of the trip.

Once back, I consulted with Doctor Boris Chandler. As I sat in his little office, gazing at the walls, I was surprised to see a portrait of Bub McAllister. Bub had been with me in college and medical school, and had been in my wedding. I later learned that Chandler had been an intern and resident under McAllister at Presbyterian in New York City and was a great admirer of him. He said that sometime in the early 1950's, McAllister had inserted the first aortic hemograft in the United States. Chandler cured me with a cortisone shot. I did not have an infection.

At six that evening, we had a rendezvous with Adrian Hilaire, now an important figure in the Haitian Sante Publique. At our hospital he had succeeded Warren Berggren as head of our Public Health Department. He was planning health care for Haiti similar to what Rex Fendall did in Kenya.

We called on Adrian's brother, the commanding general of the army. The General showed us his house on a hillside with a great view of the sea and the mountains. He filled us in on some of his domestic arrangements: rent of $500 a month on his house, and an electric bill of $120 to $150 a month, which had to be paid in advance. He took out the electric stove and installed a charcoal burner because of the expense. Water was heated on the roof. He knew about the water problem at Mole and the police control of the stream, benefiting their own gardens to the exclusion of others. "The chief problem with most Haitians is that they are underdeveloped in the head," he told us. "They can not see the forest for the trees."

General Hilaire had another brother who ran a small restaurant and snack bar called LaNova, and a brother-in-law who was a pathologist in Switzerland. I remarked that for a doctor to be happy all he needs is to confine himself to taking care of patients. General Hilaire replied, "The same with me. I mind my own business and keep out of politics." That seemed to be how he was able to maintain his position in that outrageous country.

In a Port-au-Prince art gallery, a young man came up and asked if I was Dr. Lepreau. He said I had taken care of his father who had finally died of "oppression." This could have been asthma or tuberculosis. He said he was a friend of Dr. Leslie Sycamore, a volunteer radiologist from Hanover, New Hampshire, who came for six months at a time for several winters.

We were able to visit several other acquaintances during our visit. We met Carolyn Bradshaw for lunch one day. Carolyn, a typical Protestant missionary, was on her way back to LaPointe in the northwest. She is a dedicated nurse who runs a modest operation for children with spinal tuberculosis. She is the whole show. The children must lie flat all the time, but I don't recall which side must be up. Carolyn deplored the unwise administration of USAID in Haiti.

We took Madam Peter Malensky-Malevich to see the Oloffson show. She told us her husband had founded Tanglewood before it was Tanglewood. She knew Koussevitsky and wife very well. She was an enchanting lady and we have seen her several times over the years. Here in Haiti she was a volunteer for Sister Joan in her clinic and gift shop.

We visited Bill Hodges and his wife at Limbe. They were typical nineteenth century Baptist missionaries. After medical school Bill was in the service, then went to Japan for a year or two as a missionary. He came to Haiti to revive a dying Baptist medical mission at Limbe in the north of Haiti about forty miles short of Cape Haitian. Bill was a prodigious worker, took all comers and knew a great deal of medical science. He had

a primitive laboratory and x-rays, an occasional medical
student and many volunteers, mostly from the States. He
was well acquainted with the frailties of Haitians, knew
all about their voodoo and thought this was the main
reason that they could not take care of themselves. On
one of my visits there I performed a pyloromyotomy on a
tiny dried out infant, and coached Dr. Hodges' associate
on a similar case. Both patients did well.

On another of my visits to Limbe, Monny and I
were marooned when a nearby river flooded and trapped
us in the second story of a storehouse for two days. It
was damp and it rained constantly. The place was dirty.
When the family ate meat at a meal, they threw the bones
over their shoulders to the dogs at their back. We both
agreed that the lifestyle was not one we could live with.

Bill was active in discovering and excavating
historical sites associated with Columbus. He was
certain that he had found Guacanacaric's village, the
Indian chief who welcomed Columbus, and the site of
Fort Navidad inside the village stockade. Hodges took
me to the site on the landside of Bord Limonade, east of
the Grand Riviere du Nord. He had dug a trench across
it and had found the shaft of a well filled with charcoal
and artifacts. As Indians did not dig wells, he was
confident that this was the site of the fort that Columbus
built from the remnants of the Santa Maria at the end of
his first voyage. Columbus left 39 men there, and when
he returned a year later the fort had been destroyed and
the men killed. I went digging a few times with Bill. We
used little trowels and brushes and unearthed at least
two skeletons. I think the Christians were buried on their
backs with their faces heading eastwards towards the
resurrection.   The site remains a challenge to

archeologists because it has never been proven according
to their standards. But Hodges was sure. Along with
Kathy Deagan of the University of Florida at Gainesville,
Bill Hodges was probably one of the world's authorities
on Columbus in early Hispaniola and Spanish
settlements on the north shore.

Eventually Hodges partially retired to a house
that he built on a nearby plateau overlooking the Bay of
Acule. He was an inspiring person, knowledgeable and
indefatigable and although he received criticism from
authorities, from academics, from living room liberals or
conservatives – Bill Hodges was *there*. He died of a
massive myocardial infarction on September 16, 1995 at
his retirement home at Chateau Neuf, Limbe. Thus
ended his 37 years of service to God and the Haitian
people, which had begun on April 11, 1958 when he with
his wife and four children came to revive Hôpital Bon
Samaritan.

In 1989, fifteen years after I left Haiti, Dr. Mellon
died. Writing his obituary for the Journal of the
American Medical Association gave me an opportunity
to collect my thoughts about our stay in Haiti:

> *William Larimer Mellon, Jr. MD,*
> *founder and director of Hôpital Albert*
> *Schweitzer in Haiti, died at his home there in*
> *the village of Deschapelles on August 3, 1989.*
> *He had Parkinsonism and undifferentiated*
> *cancer for 2 years, although his mental*
> *capacity remained undiminished until a month*
> *before his death. He was 79 years old.*
> *Dr. Mellon completed his education in*
> *New Orleans, LA - college at Tulane*

*University and medical school at Tulane
University School of Medicine, earning his
medical degree in 1953. He completed a 1-year
internship at Charity Hospital followed by a 1-
year fellowship at the Ochsner Clinic, both in
New Orleans, before opening the hospital on
his 46th birthday in 1956.*

*Born on June 16, 1910 in Pittsburgh,
PA Dr. Mellon attended the Choate School,
Wallingford, Connecticut and Princeton (NJ)
University but left Princeton after one year to
work for the Gulf Oil Company. Unsatisfied
with life as a businessman he became a
successful working rancher near Rimrock,
Arizona. There he met and married Gwen
Grant Rawson who was to become his lifelong
associate in his medical career. During World
War II he served in the Office of Strategic
Services.*

*The same qualities of independence
and initiative that led him to ranching brought
Dr. Mellon to his decision to emulate Albert
Schweitzer in the alleviation of human
suffering. Intrigued by Schweitzer's writings,
he corresponded with Schweitzer, visited
Lambarene, Gabon, and in time gave up
ranching to reenter college and study
medicine.*

*Hôpital Albert Schweitzer is a modern
133-bed hospital in the Artibonite Valley, 4
hours from Haiti's capital with a commitment
to care for the 150,000 poor people of the
valley. A tolerant and liberal chief, Dr. Mellon
nevertheless insisted that his staff practice*

their craft with competence and compassion, and from the outset he attracted an international group of skilled physicians and nurses who enabled him to devote most of his time to community development. Although he delegated supervision of the hospital to his wife and a few others, he remained in control.

Music was his hobby and after a long hot day in the valley he would find relaxation playing the cello accompanied by his wife on the flute.

Dr. Mellon was a shrewd judge of people. He made his own decisions and absorbed his disappointments; as Osler might have put it, he "consumed his own smoke." Surveying for a pipeline or digging a trench with a group of Haitians, he looked, moved, and acted like the cowboy he once was. And he was magical with Haitians. Committed to their welfare, he was able to work effectively through their pervasive voodoo.

Inscribed over the hospital's entrance are Schweitzer's words, "Reverence for Life." This, together with respect for all people, was Dr. Mellon's creed. Like Schweitzer's, Dr. Mellon's faith was in his works, and his teaching was by example. Visitors who came asking the meaning of life were likely to find him in the valley where he might answer them, "Perhaps you'd help load these bags of cotton into the jeep."

He contributed to the welfare of thousands of patients. He inspired hundreds of others to share personally in that most rewarding of all actions--a commitment to a cause beyond one's self.

Mrs. Mellon survives her husband and she will remain in Deschapelles to ensure that the hospital has ongoing leadership. Also surviving are a daughter-in-law, LeGrand Mellon; three step-children, Michael Rawson, Jennifer Rawson Grant, and Ian Grant Rawson; a brother, Matthew T. Mellon and two sisters, Rachel Walton and Margaret Hitchcock.

After Dr. Mellon's death, Gwen Mellon remained in Haiti carrying on with the same devotion to her husband and the Haitians he sought to help that she had shown during his lifetime. In later years, troubled by failing vision, she could frequently be found in the hospital courtyard writing Thank you notes to donors. Gwen Grant Mellon, a remarkable and inspiring person, died on November 29, 2000, aged 89. She was buried beside her husband on the grounds of their hospital.

Our own time in Haiti was running out. My chronic cough was producing purulent sputum; a skin test for rats was strongly positive. Mimi was soon to be married and now with Jay gone, Monny and I wanted to be closer to our children. We started to make plans to return home. For me and our youngest children, Mimi and Jay, our Haitian experience was a salutary one. I am not so sure about my wife. She enjoyed herself and the domestic scene, but I know she preferred our home in Westport, Massachusetts. For me it was the best of all possible worlds: a close and simple family life, the continuing medical and surgical challenges and an opportunity to teach young doctors. It was the fulfillment of a lifelong dream that William Larimer Mellon made possible.

I thought back over all that I had seen and done since we arrived in Haiti. I had adapted readily to the experience here. Daily life is basic, uncomplicated. One's work, home, ordinary food needs, and place of worship are within a few steps. Think what that bit of geography does. We did not own a car for six of the nine years we spent in Haiti. I attempted to total the time, the money and the arrangements involved in having an automobile, and realized the freedom we gained during those six car-less years.

"Simplify, simplify, simplify" was a Thoreau injunction and a Quaker premise that was easy to accomplish in a medical missionary situation. For the daily schedule one arises at dawn, has breakfast and by walking a few hundred feet arrives at the hospital. No parking, no driveways blocked by snow, no buses, no trains. Tea time at ten o'clock at the hospital, or on the veranda, lunch at home for an hour or an hour and a half (at Hôpital Albert Schweitzer it was strictly one hour) tea at three o'clock for a few minutes, closing time between four and eight in the evening, depending on the needs of the institution. Off duty, a shower, supper at home or with colleagues, reading or writing and finally to bed. If summoned, you are with your patient within five minutes. No telephone call. A messenger knocks on your door.

The patients are very sick, and few survive past 65 years of age. There are no life-support problems because the machinery does not exist. It is often like Paul De Kruif's old book, *Men against Death.* Almost all can be significantly helped by simple medicines or surgery. Infectious disease abounds. You can give fundamental advice about hygiene and prevention. Worms, heart failure, vitamin deficiencies are all common and easily cured. A fractured arm or leg, especially with one end sticking out, is perhaps not as esoteric as a coronary artery bypass or an anterior rectal resection, but it is important to the person who has it. So is a huge abscess. And the "cost benefit," which is a popular phrase now, is enormous. A hernia that keeps a man from his field, and his family from hunger, a kidney stone, a big, benign prostate, a urethral stricture, all are basic, all are easily remedied with ordinary skills and equipment.

And what about equipment? The operating room at the Friends' Africa Mission was barren. I did a successful lobectomy there with anesthesia administered by an African who used an old Boyle's machine left over from colonial days. In Kenya, cleanliness and perhaps sterility is accomplished at the end of the schedule by wiping all moveable equipment with carbolic acid and putting it out of doors in the sun for several hours. One soon learns that one can do much with little and if one does not have the knowledge or laboratory or the equipment to handle a few complex situations, there are so many more patients out there that can be cured with what one does have. There are none of the sometimes-difficult problems involved in treating "private" patients. There are minimal committee meetings and paper work. One's activities are confined to healing the sick in the most direct and personal way.

You may be lucky, as I was at Schweitzer, to have twelve bright associates, or you may be all by yourself like David Hadley at Friends' Africa Mission. Most have auxiliary help with varying degrees of ability. Rex Fendall has written, "Properly trained and nurtured auxiliaries can multiply the doctor".

Some may ask, "Why not take care of the sick in Harlem or Roxbury or the poor white of the South?" What about eastern Kentucky, the part of Appalachia where I lived for one and a half years? Even there in an area well known for its rural poor, medical care, truly good medical care was available at no cost to the patient. I know for I gave it. In Fall River, as well, I know of no patient who could not get care if he really wanted it.

Yet in Haiti, when we turned people away from our front steps we knew they had no place else to go. We were treating people from early morning until closing, working from seven in the morning to as late as nine in the evening. We cared for as many as we could possibly handle, knowing that if we couldn't take them they had no other place to turn. The choice of who would be treated and who would be turned away fell to me, personally. I made those decisions twice a day for five years and it was one of the most difficult tasks I have ever performed.

Haitian children are hungry. The birth control movement is slow. The classic question is "Why let them live?" What about Lifeboat Ethics of Garrett Hardin and the Tragedy of the Commons, and others who say these countries and their people should be abandoned? What about the influence of a fine mission station or a great medical school like Markerere, which has been destroyed by Idi Amin? What is permanent and what turns out just the way we planned? What does it all amount to? The gospel of Jesus was delivered to an oppressed world, yet He kept on and His light still beckons through the forest of missiles and sidewinders. Ghandi's dream of a free, peaceful India occurred only after a long, bloody partition. Does this mean that he should not have tried?

In spite of the sacks of AID grain stolen off the trucks in Port-au-Prince, and those American-dug canals now choked with water hyacinths, I must fall back on the fact that I am a Quaker physician. I must hoe it out on my own compass. When I see a sick or dying person, I see God in him. I have the skills to restore him. Do I have a choice? As Mary Martin sang in *South Pacific*, "I'm stuck like a dope with a thing called hope."

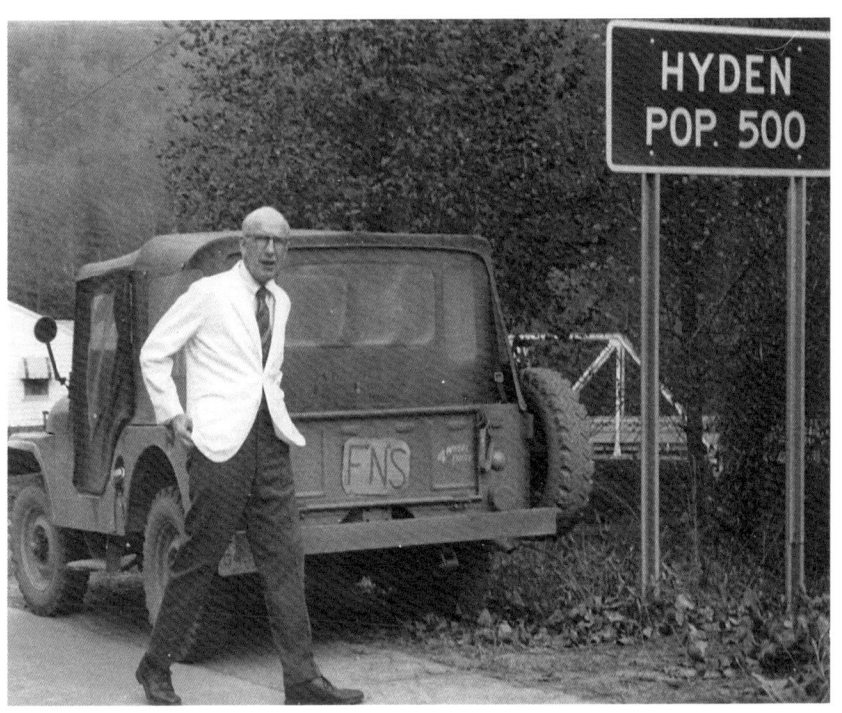

Frontier Nursing Service

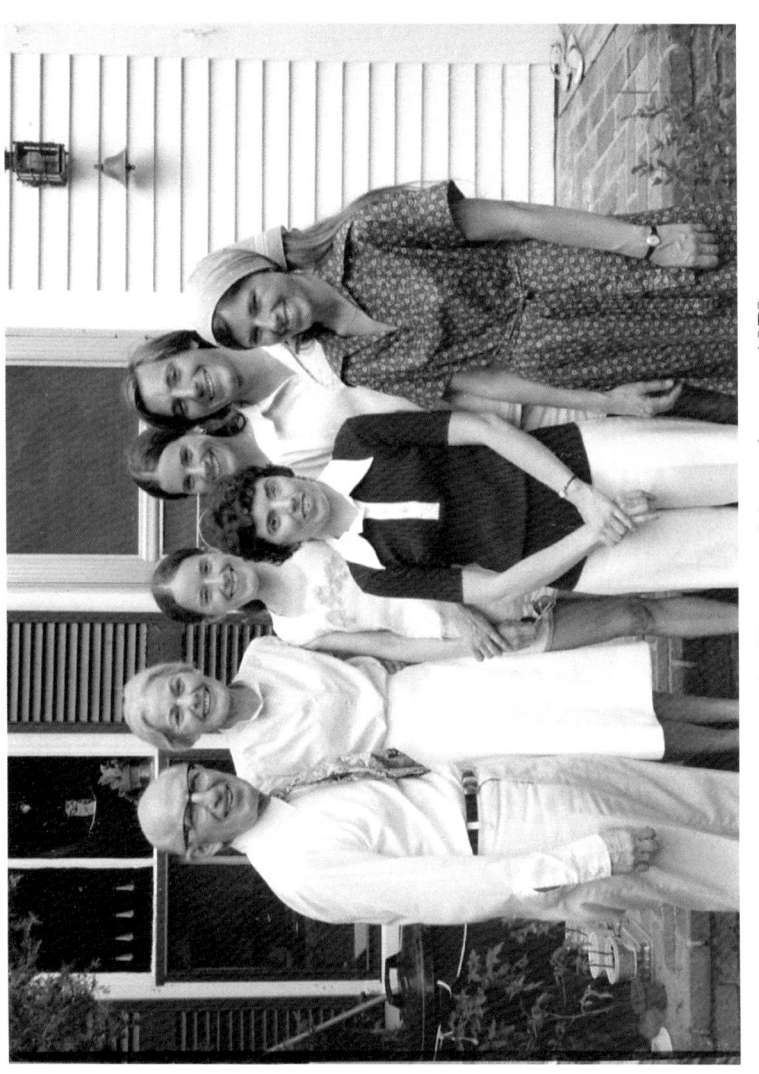

Lepreaus in Westport, Massachusetts 1979
Frank, Monny, Sue, Lucy Ann, Mimi, Jay, Judy

10

Kentucky

When I first returned to the States in 1973, I suffered reentry syndrome and even saw a psychiatrist weekly for a while. My old colleagues were kind and helpful to me, but I ended up fleeing to eastern Kentucky, true Appalachia. For two years I was the medical director and surgeon for the Frontier Nursing Service. We had a nice house on a steep hillside just a few steps from the hospital. A few years prior to our occupancy the house had slid three feet down the hill. All the plumbing had to be redone.

Mary Breckenridge of a distinguished Kentucky family had founded the Frontier Nursing Service in 1925. She had lost two husbands and two very young children, and so she devoted her life, income, and energy to people of eastern Kentucky with a particular concern for pregnant women and their children. She was remarkably successful. Her work was centered in the town of Hyden, population less than 500, nestled in the bottom of a hollow typical of the area.

Her outreach eventually comprised six or seven nursing stations scattered one day's horseback ride from each other throughout the mountains of eastern Kentucky. In these houses lived two registered nurses, at least one of whom was a certified nurse mid-wife, well trained and highly competent. At that time there were no such credentialed practitioners in the United States, so they were all imported from England.

These women did the deliveries and provided whatever health care was needed in the area. Mary Breckenridge's idea came from a similar service in the Hebrides Islands off Scotland. It was a tremendous contribution because the few roads around Hyden were mostly dirt and often muddy. There were frequent floods and no phones. Connections were made by short wave radio or courier. The one physician in the service was stationed in Hyden in a primitive wooden hospital, which was still functioning when I arrived in 1975. The physician made the rounds of the nursing stations on horseback, visiting them all over the course of seven days. He took care of cases the nurses thought too complicated and helped out in general. I had seen similar arrangements in Newfoundland and the Labrador coast when I visited the Grenfell Mission. In my time, Jeeps had replaced the horses. On one occasion I had to drive up a stream to get to my destination.

Tradition was a significant component of the FNS experience. In daily life there were frequent references to Mrs. Breckenridge and comments by a retired nurse who had worked with her and lived on the grounds. Miss Helen Browne or "Brownie," the current director, lived in the big log house at Wendover, where Mrs. Breckenridge had lived. Like her, Brownie served tea and sherry every afternoon at four. Built into the wall of the main building was a brick from Florence Nightingale's house. Another associate, Ida May January, told innumerable tales of the early days traveling in the mountains on horseback through deep snow. I have a photograph of her in a striking pose on her horse. She autographed for me Mrs.

Breckenridge's book, *Wide Neighborhoods* (Harper-Row, 1952), a story of the Frontier Nursing Service. It was a privilege to be Miss January's physician during her last days.

The Frontier Nursing Service had a remarkable record of ten thousand consecutive deliveries, mostly at home, with four deaths, two caused by blood loss, two due to cardiac disease. This accomplishment was written up and reported by the Metropolitan Life Insurance Company. These nurses were competent in handling a case, yet they were equally aware of something beyond their competence when they would call in the physician or transport the patient to an institution where there were physicians and equipment.

With the onset of World War II in 1941, the supply of English midwives ceased. That did not deter Mrs. Breckenridge. She started a school for midwives, which remains active. While I was there it was tapering off because there were not enough deliveries to sustain a school. The school subsequently made arrangements to have much of the clinical work done elsewhere, and it continues to be successful, graduating 784 certified nurse midwives in the years 1989 through 1999. The school also trains family nurse practitioners. Along with the three other physicians, my position was to train nurses, treat patients and to supply back-up for the nurses.

The following situation illustrates the nature of the Frontier Nursing Service. A call came in over the short wave radio from Ms. Blevins at her nursing station. "I am bringing in a patient who has a ruptured ectopic pregnancy." This was an emergency, as the patient could die from blood loss if not treated immediately. Soon Blevins appeared with the patient bedded on the floor of the Land Rover hooked up to an IV, and being comforted by her husband.   My interview and exam were superfluous.   The nurse had it all in hand.   Upon operating I evacuated considerable blood from the abdomen, clamped and removed the bleeding fallopian tube, closed the abdomen and reported to the husband. He listened but most of his questions were directed to the nurse-midwife, as it should have been. Blevins was the person he knew and who had acted immediately to save his wife's life.   Dr. Lepreau was just another pair of hands.

We had a few medical students from the University of Kentucky and I would have made more of that association, but the University was 150 miles away. At Hyden I was the only surgeon, although Dr. Anne Wasson, a competent, older general practitioner, did a lot of surgery and the cesareans.   I did a fair amount of complicated surgery and many cesareans but not as many as in the centers because we weren't interested in the cash register.   A board certified pediatrician was present at every cesarean, which was not the case in Fall River.

One of the pediatricians was so impressed with my speed that he had a stopwatch on me from the time I made the skin incision until I brought the baby out.   It may have been something like thirty seconds.   The operating room was the size of a large closet, complete with a wet mop and a mousetrap in the corner. Anesthesia was light, mostly local, although we did have a competent nurse anesthetist.   The equipment was adequate.   I was used to a minimal support system because of my past experience in Haiti and Africa. But daily living could be bleak.   One of the more sophisticated nurses said, "What do you say after you say hello?"

During our stay in Kentucky, we planned a rendezvous with Monny's friends, Kenny and Cleveland Rea from Pittsburg. We were to cover a wide spectrum from the elegant affluence of Kentucky thoroughbred country to the Abby of Gethsemane where men lived in silent obedience to God. In Lexington we visited Keenland Farms and racetrack as well as Calumet Farms, where eligible colts were auctioned for figures sometimes close to a million dollars. We also saw cemeteries for famous horses where only the head, hooves, and heart were interred because there was scant room for anything else. The husband of Mary Bradish, one of our nurses, was a groom at Clairborne or Calumet. He gave us a complete exposure to thoroughbred racing. I have a photo of Monny patting Secretariat who had just been retired and was now out to pasture. The owners hoped to make handsome stud fees in the five figures, but at the time of our visit he had done nothing but eat grass. The animals, both thoroughbred racers and trotting horses, lived in air-conditioned stalls. To prevent the males from defying all obstacles to get at the mares, they were kept in pastures with strong fences well away from the mares. We were shown a large room with padded walls where the principals got boisterous during the procreation act. A seller's fee of $600,000 isn't too much, nor is a stud fee of $15,000.

We stayed at Shakertown, a Williamsburg-like restoration of one of the earliest Shaker settlements dating from around 1800. The stone buildings were rectangular like the old Fall River mills, and the interiors unadorned. This was a communal and celibate society whose members were dedicated to labor and simplicity in the service of God. It was a lovely restoration. About an hour away to the west and south of Louisville is the Cistercian Abbey of Our Lady of Gethsemane. It had its own post office: Trappist, Kentucky. There is nothing else there. Early on a Sunday morning, we set out for the Abbey going through the closest town on the map, Bardstown, where Stephen Foster wrote "My Old Kentucky Home," one of more than a hundred songs that he completed. He died of alcoholism in the Bowery of New York City.

We had had no breakfast, so at a roadside pump with a tiny, tired lunch counter we had a stale doughnut and weak coffee. From there we departed contemporary U.S.A and took a side road without signs through the countryside to the monastery. It sits with its courtyard alone in the fields with a few trees immediately around it. A cemetery dating back to its founding in 1848 is outside the grounds. Thomas Merton wrote a good history of it titled *The Waters of Siloe*. Founded by French members, it is the oldest Cistercian Abbey in the United States. As we sat in the balcony we could view the impressive interior. The floor was flagstone, the walls white, the wooden stalls the monks sat in and the wooden beams that supported the ceiling were a natural color. The windows were high and narrow but large enough to flood the building with light which came through the multi-paned windows fitted with glass of white, yellow, various shades of tan and perhaps some gray, but oddly, no reds, blues or oranges.

After a worldly life in Europe and the United States, Thomas Merton entered the Abbey on December 10, 1941, at the age of 26. Within the Abbey, he was known as Father Louis. He tells his story in his book, *The Seven Story Mountain*. To the world he continued to be known as Thomas Merton, a prolific writer on religious subjects, solitude, and the contemplative life. His theme was complete submission and oneness with God. Merton resembles the Quaker, Thomas Kelley. The notable exception was that Kelley was much in the world, although not of it, while Merton in the last years of his life lived as a hermit in a building outside the monastery. One might put the question here, "Who is the truest servant of God?" Is it he who lives in solitude as a hermit or in a cloister, who prays, works in the fields, makes cheese and fruitcake as many do? Or, followers like Thomas Kelley who taught young men and women, or Sister Joan Margaret who spent three hours a day on her knees praying, the rest the day conducting the only school for the lame and the blind in all of Haiti?

Twenty-seven years after he entered the monastery, twenty seven years to the day, on December 10, 1968, after addressing a religious conference near Bangkok, Thailand, Merton was found dead in his hotel room, a corner room overlooking the harbor, with a stand-up electrical fan across his chest. In *Conjecture of a Guilty Bystander*, published two years before his death, he said, "I think I may soon die although I am not yet old. I was walking toward the center without knowing where I was going. Suddenly I come to a dead end on a height looking at a great bay, an arm of the harbor."

On my return to Hyden, Kentucky, I spoke enthusiastically of our trip to Gethsemane. Lucille Lebeau, R.N., whose family lived in New Bedford, Massachusetts, was one of my listeners. She had spent five years with a Catholic nun in a remote mission in

Brazil surrounded by jungle. Their supervising priest had received a letter from a fellow monk at Gethsemane written the day after Merton's funeral. Lucille showed it to me and I made a photocopy. It was written on onionskin, poorly typed and obviously done in haste, the kind of letter one would sit down and bang out on a typewriter to a friend with no thought of composition-- just the news and thoughts as they came to mind. I include it here because of its intimate description of Merton.

Abbey of Gethsemani
Trappist, Kentucky
December 17, 1968

Dear Friend:
    We buried Father Louis (Thomas Merton) yesterday, December 17, out in back of our Monastery church, on a slope under a cedar in full view of the wooded hill he loved. Odd, for it just struck me as a type; this, that he should be buried there, where there is no wall to obstruct the view, but right out in the open where you can see the country in all the beauty of its surroundings. Fitting.
    The funeral was at 3:30 in the afternoon. The rite was joyous – no other word will do. It was pretty near dark when we got to putting him in the ground. There were about 40 concelebrants. The archbishop was there, but he did not wish to function – he said it was for us. There were quite a few guests in the nave, invited ones, representative of the world in which Fr. Louis operated. Writers, poets, artists, peace people, nuns, priests, plain people. He died in a far-away land in the mist of concern for the monastic life in the East.

His death was confused. I mean we are not really sure what he died of: heart attack, accident with the electric fan? But rest content with the verdict that it was accidental death. There was some talk of an autopsy in the early confusion — imagine trying to arrange something like that on a phone to Bangkok! And that slowed up his return. There were frustrating delays and he got here just in time for his funeral! The coffin was not opened, so it turned out that I was right when I saw him leave and said to myself, "we will never see him again . . . " Father J. Eudes (our medical man) looked at him in Louisville. He is the only one buried in a coffin in our cemetery. Which is like him! One of those typical monsters you'd think were turned out in the shops of Metro-Goldwyn-Mayer. The readings from the book on Jonah in the Mass were not impropriate . . . There was the whale with our Fr. Louis inside. Father Daniel Walsh, who was the man who first spoke to him of Gethsemane, preached a good homily and kept it sober and dignified. It all went well and it was all rich in significant things for all of us. There was a Mozart interlude while the priests got out of their vestments (for the burying) and it sat well on the heart . . .

I do not know how to summarize the man; the thought is not even decent! Except to say that he was a contradiction. He lived at the center of the Cross, where the two arms meet. Maybe you could say, at the heart of life. And my guess is that at no other place is contradiction reconciled. He was a problem to many. Here also. And this is the reason for the problem: I mean the terrifying tensions the man endured with a kind of courage that only the power of God made possible. I kept feeling when close to him: God is near. And to be near God is to be near something at once wonderful and terrible. Like fire. It burns. People were forever trying to get out of the spot he made for them (by his simply being what he was) by putting him into some category or other and then making him stay there – about as good as bottling a fog! For the task was impossible. They could decide he is a "monk" and this is what a monk should do. Then they would expect him to do it. And he wouldn't. Couldn't. Or hermit? Very well. This is what a hermit is – and then they would see if he was being a good hermit. And he would not be! And so on. In everything.

The only way I could live with the man was to love him whole, as he was, with all his contradictions, and I think this is the way he loved me. For he was as merry a man as I have known. Yet he had depths of sadness it were best not to mention. He loved the monastic life, yet lived in a style of his own. He had a real love for the solitary life, and yet no one around here has his kind of love for people, for the world God made. He was above everything trivial and petty. And yet he kept up with everything and knew all that was going on. He could be as tough as any man with recognizable guts. And yet he was a gentle and tender as a child with a bird. He could be flippant and airy, but he could also freeze you with the intensity and ardor he felt. He had the jaunty walk of a man in his 20's, but I do not know many with the sense of compassion that he had. He loved his Monastery, yet was critical of its foibles and foolishness. He would argue and plead with his Abbot the way a shrewd lawyer would argue for a lost cause. Yet he was obedient to the core of his being. And his obedience was tested time and time again. And found pure. Pure. I cannot go on – You do not get this kind of man from the hands of God very often. He is living witness to God! To God's love for Gethsemane, for the monastic life, for the Church, our land, the world. Praised be God in His saints forever and ever. AMEN

(Ass. Matthew Kelty)

Before his conversion, Merton had summered and partied with Lloyd Goodrich in Little Compton, Rhode Island, along with Reginald Marsh and other rogues. Goodrich was a notable figure in the art world and published a coffee table book on his friend, Edward Hopper, and a beautiful two-volume set on Thomas Eakins, copies of which he autographed for me. When Goodrich became a patient of mine, he was semi-retired and spent most of the year in Little Compton. I liked to see him because he was a storehouse of information on American art and artists. He had been Director at the Whitney Museum of American Art from 1958 to 1968. He invited Monny and me to the first appearance of his Eakins biography held at his house in Little Compton in the early evening. It was a small neat affair with mostly slim, older women artists in their little black dresses wearing a bit of elegant jewelry. The Goodrichs were a lovely couple who collaborated in his life of work.

~

I do not know the correct adjective to describe the culture of eastern Kentucky except to use the broad and prejudiced term Appalachia. So I will simply relate what I saw in my years there from 1974 to 1976. Here some counties were "dry," some were not. Unemployment and welfare were high. The source of income was the waning soft coal mining industry and lumbering. Indeed the official post office was Thousand Sticks, meaning trees. Strip mining and long wall mining were the cheapest ways to get at the coal and proved destructive of the landscape, leaving huge scars on the hillsides and bare mountain tops. Abandoned automobiles, refrigerators, and washing machines filled the streams.

Was this soft coal mining a factor in causing black lung disease? Hard coal with silica is well known to cause debilitating pneumoconiosis. However, soft coal without silica blackened the lungs but may not have been a cause of respiratory distress. I think heavy cigarette smoking was the culprit. But the miners, aided by a powerful congressman named Perkins who needed to be reelected every two years, and, above all, the lawyers made it almost automatically an industrial compensable malady. A friend, Mr. Fortney, was a healthy 75 year-old man who had been in the mines since age 11 when he guided the donkeys pulling the coal-laden cars to the portal. He had never smoked. Black lung disease remains controversial.

There are few accidents in well-run mines. The majority of accidents occur in small operations where the owner of a hill digs into it without proper and safe construction. I went into the mines four times. Two of them, I remember, were well run, one by the Bethlehem Steel Company. I was a mile or so into the earth on the man cars where one cannot sit up but must lie back. In the mines, three faces were worked simultaneously. At one, there was a shooter who drilled holes three feet apart and three feet deep into the face of the coal seam. The holes were stuffed with dynamite, and then connected with wires to an instrument around a corner. When ready, the operator pushed the plunger down yelling "Fire, Fire" and the face of loose coal came tumbling down.

The face might be anywhere from four to eight feet high. The shooter would move on to another face

and repeat the procedure. He was followed by a piece of
equipment similar to a huge dust pan which, with the
assistance of spiked rollers, picked up the loose coal and
threw it back into the cars to be brought out to the portal.
After the initial drilling, dynamiting and scooping up the
coal, the roofers came in. A roofer drills holes in the rock
above and into those he inserts a long, jointed iron rod
maybe six feet long with expansion bolts on the end. The
proximal end has an iron plate eighteen inches in
diameter designed to hold the roof up. There are many of
these. Then the whole sequence resumes. It was
arranged so that each man was always occupied going
from one face to another with no face in waiting. At the
mines, I learned that John L. Lewis used to agitate for
portal-to-portal pay. The portal is where one enters the
mine from the outside world. Lewis successfully
achieved pay for the miner from the time he entered the
portal through the return trip to the surface.

I found a strong family bond in this part of
Kentucky. There were no nursing homes in Leslie
County. The sick, the physically or mentally disabled,
were part of the family, often ensconced in a cluttered
central room used for living, dining and kitchen
activities. Washing often hung out on the porch. On my
house calls I repeatedly witnessed the strength and
bonds within these families. I recall one visit where the
patient, an older man, sat in a corner of the room with a
catheter draining into a bottle at his side. His wife was
stirring around and their 50-year-old daughter was
sitting there. I engaged her in conversation, and asked
where she came from. "London," she replied. I was
surprised as London was about 100 miles away. On

inquiring how she came to be way over here, she answered, "It's my turn."

This was also a gun culture. My scrub nurse carried a derringer in her purse and moon shiners were still making illegal whiskey. One morning, as the nurses came in from their trailers or small houses on the periphery of Hyden, they said, "There were a lot of fireworks on Asher's Branch last night." I asked, "What do you mean?" They replied, "There were a lot of gun shots because the Feds were raiding a still." And this was in 1975. Also repeated trespassing, despite several warnings by the owner, could result in a shooting, sometimes fatal. A perfunctory trial exonerated the owner because the trespasser had been warned.

Frontier Nursing Service was my first consistent exposure to alcoholism and particularly Alcoholics Anonymous. "J", a lady of 55 who was part of a wealthy Cleveland industrial family, was in recovery and actively supportive of the Nursing Service and the local Alcoholics Anonymous. Although not a nurse, she provided financial, personal, and psychological support to both. I became friendly with "C" whose hernia I repaired. "C" pushed cartons around in the back of the only grocery store in Hyden and he, too, was in recovery. He took me to A.A. meetings in the basement of the Presbyterian Church. I probably attended two thirds of the meetings and since I knew nothing about alcoholism, I was smart enough not to speak.

Near the end of my stay in Hyden I began to realize why the members were so pleased when I appeared. The alcoholics felt themselves at the bottom of the social ladder, and were pleased when a square person with some standing in the community, at least in their opinion, would be willing to sit with a few "bums" for a couple of hours once a week. I may not have interpreted it properly, but that's what I think. They always asked when I didn't show up, "Where were you last week, Doc? We missed you."

That was the beginning of my experience with alcoholics and later with drug addicts which I took up with much vigor in Fall River. Edwin Jaffe, a Yale alumnus and president of J & J Corrugated Box, Ricky Alpert and I started the Stanley Street Detoxification and Rehabilitation Center, now called SSTAR. Ed's father, Myer Jaffe, was a philanthropist who helped found Brandeis University. Mrs. Alpert was a psychiatric social worker in Fall River, whose husband had served as a Marine in the bloody fighting at Okinawa or Iwo Jima. The building that houses the rehab center is now named after me.

11

Later Years

In the years following our return from Kentucky, we settled in Westport and caught up on life in the States. My children were scattered across the country: Jay was in Utah, Judy, Suzy, and Lucy were in Rhode Island, and Mimi was in Indiana. We found a house on River Road in Westport and started to remodel it to our tastes. We took time to enjoy several vacations together. Monny and I completed a cross-Canadian train ride from Montreal or Toronto to Vancouver, British Columbia. My penciled notes indicate that we made a trip to Utah to visit with Jay and his family.

> *Arrived in Salt Lake City on Friday, the thirteenth about 8:00a.m. after a train ride from Seattle; we had not slept much because of the noise from the rails. Jay met us at the station in a small rattling unlicensed Land Rover.*
>
> *We made a trip over the mountain near Bingham where we saw mountains, yes, mountains of slag from one of the world's largest open pit copper mines. As one peered down from the top, the bulldozers and trucks looked like tiny toys. We saw several men on top near us with their dirt bikes and one with a pickup going up and down the hill. The pick-*

up driver had a dog that was three quarters wolf and one-quarter malamute that was known to be wonderful with children. He was gentle with Frank, but a few weeks earlier, the owner had seen him take the neck out of a Doberman Pincer in thirty seconds. Later we had coffee and pastry at a unique coffeehouse called the Salt Lake Coffeehouse, bare bones, clean, coffee in huge cups, luscious pastries.

Next week Linda will go to a retreat at Ghost Ranch, a place where Georgia O'Keefe spent a few pleasant years.

Renee is a charmer. We colored. Frank is an explorer. Jay and Linda are good parents. Jay seems to adore his children and they him.

Jay took us on several trips through the canyon country of Utah. In his kayak he accompanied Monny and me down the Grand Canyon. We were in a six-person paddle raft and safely negotiated all the rapids except Crystal. The water was too high and, indeed, a guide's raft had overturned. The most exciting rapid for us was Lava. We did the Excalante Wilderness and the Burr Trail. I think it was in the latter that the canyon wall at our point of exit seemed straight up. Jay, with a big pack, skirted around to find what he thought was a good place for him to ascend, but it was too chancy for us. He threw a rope down to us at the bottom and pulled Monny up. Then, my turn. The proper technique for the person being pulled up is to keep his body perpendicular to the wall and so I was when,

*half way up, Jay called, "Hey Dad, hold it.
That's great. Nothing but you and sky. I'll
get a picture." And so he did, of his frightened
75-year-old father.*

*We went down the Middle Fork of the
Salmon and also the Main Salmon as well. We
did several hiking and self-contained camping
excursions. It was fun, always a challenge.
The stark beauty of the desert interrupted by
huge rock formations, buttes, arches, deep
canyons lined with stripes of desert tapestry,
and, at the bottom, a shallow, sparkling stream
bordered by various greenery. Marvelous!
One needs an Arthur Krock or Edward Abbey
to adequately describe its grandeur. The
small, dry, shallow bowls in the rock suddenly
show stirrings of life after a rain. A campsite
at Dead Horse Point, where the Green meets
the Colorado, or another camp at Zane Grey's
Robbers Roost, adds a romantic touch. Jay,
adventurous as always, was a careful guide,
taking pains to care for his 75-80 year-old
parents. He carried water, map, and compass.*

We returned to Haiti for a visit in March, 1979,
and stayed again at the Oloffson in the plush Lillian
Hellman Suite with its lovely furnishings and accessories,
and a private veranda. The air conditioning was a luxury
and helped to drown out the barking dogs, chickens and
other noises of the city. During our stay there, we met
Brian Donaldson, a lean fiftyish freelance photographer
who could have passed for a leathered Texas rancher.

Brian had come to photograph Al and Sue Seitz and the Oloffson. Brian was widely traveled and spent time on Guadalcanal during the war. He was drawn to Haiti because of the friendliness of the people, enjoying, just as I do, the press of crowds and the people around the iron market. He agreed to take several photos of Sue and Al for me. When he finished the photo session, I took the undeveloped film home where Penny Leuvelink Hadfield developed it.

On our next return, we went first to New York City and visited my brother, Bill, who was awaiting an aortic resection in the veteran's hospital associated with New York University. We saw him post-operatively and found him doing well. We stayed overnight in New York City at the Gramercy Park Hotel on one of the higher floors. It was lovely looking down at the streets with rows of lights on either side illuminating the softly falling snow. It reminded me of a Childe Hassam painting. Conditions worsened during the night. The next morning, driving a small green convertible Carmen Ghia, we arrived at Kennedy Airport in a blizzard. This was a major storm. We pulled into a Holiday Inn and were snowbound for three days.

We eventually left Kennedy Airport via National and arrived at Miami International Airport, spending a lot of time in lines, and facing several delays. To pass the time we walked around Miami Beach, which was deserted. Monny and I were not spring chickens but we looked like high school students compared to the people walking on the streets in Miami Beach. We purchased pastrami and smoked salmon for Al Seitz at the Oloffson. Finally on the third day, after two false starts, we left.

Once at the Oloffson we were shown to Chambre B, a familiar suite.   It was nostalgic to visit that place again where I had entertained Monny on her first night in Haiti. Our room had a small porch with flowers and overlooked the swimming pool. We relaxed with dinner and drinks and socialized with other visitors, among them Hal Holbrook, the frequent impersonator of Mark Twain. At midnight we went to the El Rancho where we had coffee and danced to a great orchestra.   We practically closed up the place around 1 a.m. We came back to Room #117 at the Oloffson, the Anne Bancroft suite, which had several rooms ending in a balcony. There I took some pictures of my gorgeous wife in her elegant dressing gown.

On arriving at the hospital, we met with Dr. Mellon and other old friends and passed several nostalgic hours. We had dinner with Muller, and went with him in a new air conditioned Volvo to L'escale, the small tuberculosis sanatorium with its open windows high up on the walls, to prevent the spirits from spitting on the patients. We toured the hospital: no patients with tetanus, the medical ward was down, but much malaria. Dr. Mellon gave me some cherry seeds from Lambarene, and I still wonder what I did with those seeds.

As we gassed up at the carre-four with a hand pump from a drum, we saw Archelus. I had performed bilateral lung resections for tuberculosis on Archelus several years earlier. I recalled that he went completely derange' post operative. I have a Kodachrome of him sitting on top of two chairs close to the ceiling of Ward 1. He couldn't read or write but I subsequently employed him to collect sputa in front of the hospital. I garbed him in a surgeon's gown, gave him a cap and a mask so he could feel important working for the big doctor. He was installed outside my office in the courtyard in front of the hospital with sputum cups. When I came through the door of the hospital about five minutes of seven, he'd have several people lined up with the sputum cups, exhorting them to cough saying "Ptussez, ptussez nu." He collected the sputa and took it up to Rick Kueneman who looked for tubercle bacilli under the florescent microscope. Rick had a diagnosis in a few minutes instead of waiting for the standard old-fashioned Ziehl-Neelsen stain. Archelus provided a real service; he was paid a pittance, did a good job, and acquired importance.

We planned to go to Mole St. Nicholas and stopped at Gonaives. Our driver had scabies and we got him taken care of with medicine from the pharmacy. The trip over bad rocky roads was a long one. We saw the salt works set up on the flat dry coastline of Baie de Henne. The salt is made from the seawater, which is encouraged to flow into a man-made enclosure, which is subsequently closed. Upright sticks are placed here and there as nidi for salt deposits. At Baie de Henne we stopped in the blackest of night and heard a voice, "Dr. Lepreau?" We were at the house of Mme. LaBelle Chorro, Madame LaBelle's daughter. Several years ago Madame LaBelle had a uterine carcinoma and she recognized my voice because we had got some of the latest magic medicine from the Lying-In Hospital in Boston to take care of her. I hadn't heard of or seen this patient for at least five years when we were up this way once before in Anse Rouge. We stopped at the house of a grateful patient who insisted on giving us lunch in the middle of a boiling hot day, preparing her one chicken that was tied to a post in the barren yard. We saw Dr.

Payel, a recent medical school graduate who was assigned to country clinics for one or two years. He gets $125 a month.

Mole St. Nicolas, a modest headland, was sighted by Columbus on December 5, 1492, and named after the feast day of St. Nicolas.   Monny and I had visited John Breslin and his medical clinic before.   I filled in at the clinic, doing some minor surgery.   I found a lot of scabies, and a new tuberculosis case with a severe rectal stricture due to a lymphopathia venereum diagnosed by the Frei test. I saw a new eight-month-old child with pneumonia and marked dehydration treated with a solution made up using 1000 cc water, two tablespoons of sugar, half a teaspoon of salt and a quarter teaspoon of baking soda. I subsequently acquired *Where There is No Doctor* by David Werner from the Hesperian Foundation (P.O.Box 1692, Palo Alto, California 94302).   This is a great book and I sent one to Father Breslin.   I performed a Cesarean section on a patient I had treated for tuberculosis at HAS. She was full term in labor with the fetus lying crossways in the uterus, one arm hanging out of the vagina.   I do not remember the outcome of the fetus but even with Breslin's meager facilities I was able to save the mother's life.   The next day I drained an osteomyelitis of the iliac crest in a child. Breslin used me as a helper and consultant, but in general he knew a lot of medicine and provided the only medical care in this forlorn and desolate area.

Monny and I took time to go to the beach, a beautiful beach with Monny looking glamorous in a white robe. We walked the settlement where we passed a tiny gambling "casino" with two card tables, several casks of Claren, a strong rum, and a crap table run by the deputy. There was a military post there manned by three men. The commandant had control of the only water in the place, a tiny stream, and he made sure his garden got most of it.

I have so many recollections of Father Breslin, a slender white American with a strong Brooklyn accent, who, I think, was a member of the Montfortian Associates. When we first saw him, he was covered with grease and getting down from a windmill of his making to provide a bit of electricity for his small facility on this barren landscape. All was hot, hot and dry, very dry. He was glad to see us and was a gracious host, sharing his rolls and thin chicken soup through which one could see the chicken's foot, claws and all.

After Breslin cleaned off the grease, we sat on the porch overlooking the ocean and had a rum and lemonade, then the chicken soup supper. He left afterward to conduct church services, and Monny and I walked over to observe. It was a black night. The small church was illuminated by one Coleman lantern, which made sharply contrasting black shadows and white light over the black faces, the white walls, and the supporting posts. Then from the left of the altar appeared Father Breslin in his white surplice. He read from the Bible, which was illuminated by a candle carried by a boy at his side. He continued with the mass and the Stations of the Cross.

Later that night he took me on rounds in his hospital, which had been a nunnery, built in 1906, and now an empty shell with a dirt floor. Patients and their families were in clusters scattered around directly on the floor or on thin fiber mats. A water bottle and a pot for food were all they had. Candles illuminated some of the sick. Father Breslin spoke to each group and explained their condition to me. All were serious but one he considered hopeless was an eight-year-old girl with advanced lymphoma with many nodes in the neck, axilla, and groin but no splenomegaly. I knelt down to examine her. I needed more light and Father Breslin set the kerosene lantern beside her. The lymphadenopathy was evident but nearby were 4-5 mm black linear scars. Her skin was light as is often the case in severely ill Haitian children. The black scars were easily noted. I asked the mother about the scars. "Oh, they were once bubos just like the ones you see now. They broke open and a lot of pus came out." With confidence, but trying to be modest, I told Father Breslin the lumps were tuberculosis and, if he treated her promptly, she would be cured. I was sure of it. I wish all my medical encounters could be so dramatic.

Before leaving, we talked at length about Voodoo and Christianity. Breslin thinks the nation is steeped in Voodoo and there is no hope for them to become Christians. He said, "Haitians have no concern for community good, no thought for the future. They are dishonest, need constant supervision and threats of discipline must always be present."

In Port-au-Prince I talked with Jim Sanders, an energetic, able lay person about forty years old from the Midwest who was a major co-founder of Grace Hospital for Children with Tuberculosis in Haiti. He was the first superintendent. One day he interviewed me in depth on the porch of the Oloffson about the specifics of running a hospital. He was for real and made a great contribution. I think he remained at his post for eighteen months.

We had a fascinating conversation at supper with Susan Malensky-Malevich at the Convent. She told us in detail about the idealistic beginnings, the tribulations, and the bare survival of Simons Rock College in Great Barrington, Massachusetts. Betty Hall, the daughter and heir of Thomas Blodgett, the Chicle fortune man, founded Simons Rock in 1964. Betty Hall had been the highly successful headmistress of Concord Academy. My niece, Louise Jackson Whitney, has a son William Jackson, who has taught at Simons Rock College for twenty years. Susan catered all the meals there for seven years.

We had first met Susan at the Convent in Haiti a few years before, and subsequently spent a weekend at her permanent home in Lenox. She turned out to be the widow of a Russian noble of the old regime. Her house was crammed with imperial memorabilia. Now she makes her living by catering expensive functions. Monny, Jay, Linda Lepreau, and I were finishing luncheon at her house when the servant brought finger bowls — unrecognized as such by Linda, Jay and me. The bowl sat on a doily on a decorative plate, and on the still liquid floated a tiny flower. Was it some exotic dessert? We waited. Monny, of course, knew, and we followed her lead, rinsing our fingers in the bowl.

Susan told us about Bishop Voeglie's return to Haiti, how pleased he was, then disappointed, that he was not consulted or asked to preach from time to time. He was recognized a few times. He sold his small but lovely house at Montrouis for $150,000 and returned to the States. No property in Haiti can be left to a relative who does not live in Haiti. He apparently made the local church unhappy because he did not resign his post when

he first left Haiti. Because of this they could not appoint
a new bishop.

Mary Ellen Mack, who was there taking pictures
for *People* magazine, told us some fascinating stories. She
has just returned from six weeks in India. This was her
eleventh trip, spent taking photos of Mother Theresa to
illustrate a major story for *Life* magazine. Mother
Theresa, she says, is a happy, vibrant person who was
recently in Haiti to dedicate a home for the terminally ill.

I visited the Little Sisters of Charity on Rue St.
Martin, a new 50-75 bed cement facility for homeless
tuberculosis adults who get PAS-INH streptomycin. No
Thiazena. There are three Indian nuns and two French
nuns here, all resulting from Mother Theresa's visit. We
also went to Kenscoff, almost to Furcy, and stopped at
the Baptist Mission, which was flourishing with much
activity, especially agricultural work.

Our return to Haiti in March 1990 was our last,
and our feelings were mixed. For me, returning to Haiti,
seeing and working with John Breslin, catching up with
Bill Hodges and seeing his latest archaeological digs,
getting to see Sister Joan and her work – all were
important. Living and working in Haiti had been a great
experience for me, but I could see that it was in the past
now. We found Haiti hot, and our social obligations
numerous and tiring. Monny had expressed the desire to
see more of the U.S.A.   We spent one of our last days
there sitting around the pool at the Oloffson.   We
chuckled at a young child's observation, "You are
swimming with your clothes on." she said to Monny.
The pool was decorated with numerous ladies in skimpy
bikinis, while Monny wore a modest swimsuit with skirt
and briefs beneath.

~

Recently, I resumed work on the story of my life. I reread the letters that I had written to my parents, letters that started during my college years and continued throughout our absences from the States and into the 70's. I started to think back over some of the momentous occasions which I had lived through and what I had been doing when they transpired. Here are a few:

November 11, 1918, Armistice Day: I was six years old and standing on a table in an expensive hotel dining room in Washington, D.C. while my father led the room in singing the Marseillaise like Laszlo did in Casablanca.

May 21, 1927, Lindbergh's transatlantic flight: I was in my seat looking out of a classroom window in the Hastings-on-Hudson public school. I was 15 years old.

April 12, 1945, Franklin D. Roosevelt's death: I was sitting beside Dr. Louis Byars as he drove to his office from the Barnes Hospital in St. Louis where I had spent the morning watching him and his colleagues operate.   They were the best plastic surgeons in the country and the best technicians at Barnes.   They were often called upon by other specialists to help in difficult situations.   I saw one of them, Dr. Frank McDowell, take a freehand graft intact from the posterior upper thigh to well into the calf.   I was spending part of a month in St. Louis as an exchange resident surgeon from Yale on the chief's service, Dr. Evarts Graham.   He had contributed so much to mitigate the high mortality of influenza in World War I by the proper use of closed pleural drainage. He was also one of the first, back in the early 1940's, to link cigarette smoking to lung cancer. He ran his service in the old Geheimrat system. He was a rapid and rough technical surgeon. As I watched him do a lung resection, a fairly large bleeder appeared in the field. His assistant was stopped from clamping it by Graham's words, "Get away from that capillary."

November 22, 1963, John F. Kennedy's death: I was in my long white coat entering Room 208 of the old Truesdale Hospital to visit a patient. Room 208 was a large room on the second floor of the hospital reserved for special patients.

July 20, 1969, First man to walk on the moon. Neil Armstrong was the United States' first astronaut on the moon. Dr. Harold May, my surgical colleague, and his wife Aggie were having supper at our house in Haiti. We went to the open area by the swimming pool and watched a bright moon.

12

Thoughts on Medicine and Surgery

In the practice of surgery, the aims and values which I tried to emulate were the quiet manner of David Cheever and the gentleness of his hands, the careful handling of tissue by William Halsted of Johns Hopkins. From Gervase Connor, the martinet resident surgeon at Yale, I learned meticulous post-operative care of my patients. Excepting an obvious terminally ill cancer patient, Connor would never let a patient die from a surgical complication. He would have the whole place up all night, but he would be there too. His philosophy became mine and remained so. I still feel his rapier look because of an omission of mine. There is no rationalizing. There are no excuses. Ultimately, no matter what anyone else says, once you have made an incision in a patient, you are the responsible person. You cannot pass that obligation off to anyone else.

Here are aphorisms that I posted in my operating room.

Complications are made in the Operating Room.

If an operation is difficult, you're not doing it properly.

Robert E. Gross

Gross was the first to ligate a patent ductus, which he discarded in favor of division. He later became the chief of surgery at the Boston Children's Hospital.

Other quotes that I posted above the scrub sink came from Ephraim McDowell, who, in 1823, wrote to Dr. W. C. Galt, the referring physician:

> *This case proves that appearances in surgery are often deceitful, and that while the taper of life continues to burn, although it may be faint, there is yet hope . . .*
>
> *. . . my incisions were made so free and extensive that I have always performed every part of this operation by sight.*

McDowell performed the first successful removal of an ovarian tumor on December 25, 1809, in Danville, Kentucky.

Patients are often referred to surgeons by other doctors, family practitioners, medical men, or other surgeons. But the surgeon has to make up his own mind whether surgery is indicated. It all comes under the general heading of judgment and ethics. He has to make a judgment on his own. Is this the right operation for this patient? Will he stand it? Will it really bring him sufficient years of useful life? The referring doctor may insist, but the surgeon must follow his own assessment.

The attitude of some surgeons is that they are merely technicians and must do whatever the referring physician or specialist recommends. The surgeon must know enough general medicine to make up his own mind and be confident enough to refuse. If the referring physician or the family insist on an operation which you think is not in the best interest of the patient, don't make a capital case out of it. Just say pleasantly, "Then you should see someone else." and give them a few names.

If, after a few years in training, you do not have reasonable hands then change your career. Your world will not come to an end. But if you persist in operating with a pair of hams, instead of hands, good skillful hands, your patient will come to an end along with your own career. One of my colleagues and best friends in medical school was a saint. He was smart, Phi Beta Kappa, and Alpha Omega Alpha. He was bright and studied hard. He wrote papers, did good research, became chairman of the department of surgery in an important medical school, but he could never learn to operate. He was finally moved over and was devastated. It is often difficult for an individual to estimate his own competency but a surgeon can tell by watching other people and assessing how their hands work.

Post-operatively, the surgeon has continuing responsibility. Other people may consult. One of the current traps is for the surgeon to back off and yield to advice or care from others when his patient is not doing well. He should take all the advice and consultations into consideration but ultimately he must make the decision.

The surgeon must know enough general medicine to participate in pre-op decisions: he must know anatomy, he must be dexterous, and he must be able to make decisions by himself. There is something called the loneliness of the operating room. It is there at 3 a.m. when the surgeon has a three year old child in front of him, abdomen open, blood pouring from somewhere, truly pouring out. There is no other doctor in the room and the frightened parents in the waiting room fully expect their child to come through surgery and return to normal. What do you do?

I think back to my professor of surgery at Yale, Dr. Samuel C. Harvey, a cool, Olympian figure. I have seen Harvey follow the advice he gave us. When in trouble, put a big pack, like a Turkish towel, in the abdomen and hold it for ten minutes by the clock. Hold it yourself, or have a nurse or assistant hold it while you wash your hands in the washbasin. This allows you to collect your thoughts, get your feet on the ground, and cool off while the blood flow is arrested. By the time you pull the pack out, the finite site of bleeding may be visible and you can correct it with the proper procedure.

Let's say you do that, you put in the big pack, and you wait for the ten minutes, which always goes by so slowly. You tell everyone to be alert, to pull gently on the retractors, have the suction ready, the intravenous or blood running. You gently remove the superficial pack, slowly, slowly and suddenly, whoosh, a Niagara of blood pours out. But within that tiny second you see that it is coming from a torn spleen in the left upper quadrant of the abdomen. You put a hand in, pull it out of the wound and apply two clamps. The bleeding stops. You put the stitches in the artery and vein, the spleen is in the pan, everybody gives a sigh of relief. Someone even makes a wise crack.

You sew up the wound but not the superficial skin. No stitches, but paper steri strips, because this is a female child and you want to minimize the scar. You drop your mask, take off your gloves, get rid of the bloodied operating gown and go out to tell the mother and father that there child is fine. Color returns to their cheeks. They put their arms around you but you don't know what to say. Best to say nothing, which is a basic, in talking with patients. If you don't know what to say, stick to the essentials only. "All will be well, there is no problem. Of course, it is a week or so for convalescence, but I think everything is going to be all right."

Now, is this an ego trip? Of course, it's an ego trip. You, Frank J. Lepreau, saved a life, restoring a child to her family. Although you have been scared to death for a while, your hands were what did it. It's like climbing Mount Everest every day. That's fine, of course. But what if you must go out in the hall and tell the worried parents that Mary, their Mary, is dead. Some situations are clear right from the beginning, but in others the chances may have been slim and you've told the family so, told them you would give them your very best but you weren't all that optimistic. There is that borderline case. The patient is sick, yes, very sick, but not hopeless.

Good judgment is constantly required. Should you have waited until you had blood running in a vein before operating or should you have waited until a transfusion had brought the pressure up to normal? Did you wait too long and miss the golden few minutes? Resuscitation methods take time and by the time you decide to cut, is it too late? Let's say it is a juvenile diabetic, risky at anytime. Should you give her glucose? Or give her insulin? Get another chemistry panel? How close to a normal blood sugar is close enough while the clock is ticking? Are you afraid of malpractice? Should you get a CT Scan to see if her spine is OK from the automobile injury? All this defines one of the major differences between surgery and any other specialty. One must make a decision with incomplete evidence. Hippocrates, 2500 years ago, wrote the following, which is inscribed on one of the major buildings of the Harvard Medical School:

> *Life is short, art is long, the occasion instant, experiment perilous, decision difficult.*

In the case of the child with the bleeding spleen, there are two ways to handle it. Stitch the spleen and stop the bleeding, a desirable move because of the immune qualities of the spleen that could minimize an otherwise overwhelming pneumococcus pneumonia in the future.

Currently, the advice is to do what you can to leave the spleen in. But with a big tear and ferocious bleeding you must make a quick decision. Should you remove it or leave it in? Which is the right scientific thing to do?

If you make the wrong decision, the child will die. Someone could second-guess you next week or next year. This child could develop a severe pneumonia and, because you took the spleen out, their malpractice lawyers are all over you. The operating room gets lonely. You look around and there is no one more experienced, more senior, than yourself. Nurses, interns and students can give you advice, but you have to make the ultimate, lonely decision. That is part of the business. If you are going to be a surgeon, that's what you have to expect.

Another case report on acting alone: The patient was a friend, a man with a wonderful family and a successful business, a fine person. He was in a happy second marriage after his first wife had died. He staggered into my office about ten years ago with his wife, who was younger, and a mature son, who was a socially conscious local businessman.

During a standard neurological examination, I determined that he had a major lesion in his head, most likely a brain tumor, maybe a stroke. I sent him for a CT scan that showed a mass on one side of his brain impinging on part of a vital structure. From the location of the tumor and the way it had displaced the contents of the brain, it had to be a glioma, an inoperable malignant tumor. I called a neurosurgeon for confirmation. He said, "OK. You admit him and I'll work him up."

I thought to myself: he's had a CT scan, which located the tumor anatomically; it is pressing on vital structures and is incorporating some of them. I had done the usual chest film, blood counts, and urine. What other thing was there to work up except perhaps a lumbar puncture? But, that might have precipitated a herniation of the brain into the foramen magnum at the base of the skull where the spine exits. So we had a family session and I stated my case that it was clearly inoperable, and I didn't think there was much to do in a hospital. I certainly didn't advise an operation. We all wanted a second opinion. They saw the neurosurgeon who concurred that it was inoperable and agreed with me. I treated my patient without further tests. He remained on the sun porch of his house attended by family, nuns and nurses. The family was grateful. He didn't have chemotherapy, he didn't have x-ray treatments, and he didn't have a lot of scientific torture under the guise of "modern medicine." This was a judgment call and quite a responsibility.

Many years ago while in training, Dr. Harvey dealt me a mild rebuke: I was an intern, a brand new, naïve, intern, and in those days the intern passed the instruments. The professor was on the far left, next the assistant resident and finally me. Across was the resident surgeon. The operating field was quite a distance from me but nevertheless I was expected to pass the appropriate instruments. I was green and didn't know much about the operation, but I was breaking my neck to comply. He put out his hand. I gave him a clamp but he didn't take it. I nudged the assistant resident aside, gave him another instrument, and he didn't take that. On the third try he dropped it, looked at me and said "What is your name?" "Lepreau." "Lepreau, if you are going to be a surgeon you have to learn to make up your mind." That was in 1940, more than 64 years ago. Thank heavens I made that mistake and thank heavens he looked at me and gave me the business. It saved a lot of patients' lives.

In medical school I was once in the amphitheater of the Peter Brent Brigham Hospital presenting my patient's case. I had practiced by locking myself in the john and speaking to the mirror. When my turn came I found myself standing in the middle of a wide-open space as if I were at Epidaurus with those many tiers staring down at me. I was in the pit at the Brigham with an amphitheater full of my colleagues and the first row occupied by a group of visiting elite surgeons from the East Coast hosted by Dr. William Quimby, the chairman of urology, and a heavyweight in his field. I thought I was doing pretty well when suddenly he called out, "What's your name?" "Lepreau." "Lepreau, sit down, that's muddy thinking." You can see what an impression that made on me, these many, many years later.

Robert Zollinger at the Brigham, an outstanding young surgeon, was also hard on students. I don't remember what I was doing, probably just standing around, when he said, "Come on, Lepreau. Get your hands out of your pockets and get going." Who is the more effective teacher — one who is tough or one who is gentle? I don't know. I do know the teacher should like the student. Be prepared. Know the subject. Don't fake it. We are all learning together. Be fair and be consistent.

All my professional life, from the age of twenty-six, I've been a practicing hands-on clinician. I was a general surgeon for forty-seven years until I put down the scalpel at the age of seventy-two following my last operation, the expert removal of a gall bladder followed by a smooth recovery. Along the way some surgeons stray to other careers in academia and research but most of us who are competent with our hands, who have adequate and safe judgment, and have the physical and emotional stamina to tolerate the occasional heavy stress of the operating room, just love the challenge, beginning with the first stroke of the scalpel. It's me against the world when a patient risks himself with me. I'm there with an anesthetist, maybe another physician across the table, a scrub nurse and circulating nurse, but really it's me. These people will do their best to bail me out if I falter, but if I make the wrong cut or clamp the wrong blood vessel, I'm responsible.

I can't say much about the morals and ethics of medical practice that adds anything new. It's all in the Ten Commandments and the Sermon on the Mount. The problem is that we know what we ought to do, but sometimes it's just difficult and we think impossible. Or are we just too lazy to act appropriately? I suppose the golden rule, "Do unto others as you would have them do onto you." is as good as any. The problem lies in getting an education or guidance in ethics and interpersonal relationships, no matter what religion one was brought up in. I'd say it has to come early in childhood and, in particular, from one's parents. My parents never gave me any great lectures but led by their example. Schweitzer taught by example. I believe this kind of teaching is the most effective.

I think medical school experiences solidify the good values that one was brought up with. And if the values were not taught during childhood, perhaps a good medical school education will help. I'm not speaking about the scientific aspects of it. I was strongly influenced and I still am by a succession of outstanding teachers who are long gone but whose memories persist. Let me cite a few.

Dr. Robert Green in the Department of Anatomy treated each cadaver with respect and also taught the classics in the college. Dr. Henry Jackson taught physical diagnosis with his own dynamic, didactic technique. I can still see him down there at the blackboard: one-two-three . . . that's the way it is! We loved it.

Jackson introduced me to a series of three essays by Francis W. Peabody, one of the books that influenced me most in my medical career. I still have the original copy and I've underlined many places, often referring to it. Two of the essays were most important for me. *The Care of the Patient* has become a classic. The other describes in detail how a chief should set his stamp on his under-staff and allow himself to be accessible to them, particularly to students who might be all worked up about their future. Instead of asking them to come back next week when he ordinarily sees people, he should see them immediately because they'll never get wound up enough to approach the chief again. Peabody had written that response to Warfield Longcope, chief of medicine at the Johns Hopkins Hospital and Medical School, who had written Peabody for suggestions about how to run the clinic. Much of the essay concerned the problem of full-time versus part-time clinical faculty. Peabody said, "What we want is less of the system and law that kills and more of the spirit that gives life." He died one day later of cancer of the stomach at the age of 46.

I am grateful to Dr. William Castle on how to make a diagnosis and how to apply the true scientific method. Four of us students were standing around a bed in the wards of Boston City Hospital wondering whether the female patient had a urinary tract infection. Castle muttered some mild phrase like "hell", or "damn" followed by "Let's find out". He went to a closet, got a bedpan and asked the nurse to pull the curtain and put the pan beneath the patient. The lady passed a urine specimen, he took the bedpan, and we trotted down the hall, four of us behind him, to the grungy Boston City Hospital's interns' laboratory. We put the urine under the microscope and there were the white cells. Just like John Hunter, "Don't guess. Do the experiment."

The atmosphere around the Harvard Medical School and its teaching hospitals was such that I could stop and ask the austere Edward Churchill at the Massachusetts General Hospital about lung resections.

Similarly, Elliot Cutler, Chief of Surgery at the Peter Brent Brigham Hospital, would stop as he flew down the pike with white coat flying to answer what might be a ridiculous question by a third year student. I recall one hot August afternoon in the wards of the Boston City Hospital when the Nobel Prize winner, George R. Minot, spent at least a half an hour teaching me and another student how to take a dietary history from a classic Boston City Hospital patient who had an alcohol problem.

That was in marked contrast to the three months I served on the surgical service of the Presbyterian Hospital and Columbia Medical School in New York City as a fourth year student. I had wanted to see what the rest of the world was like. On my first ward rounds I stepped up and presented my case. I had studied well the night before, boning up on the case so I knew what I was talking about. The Professor looked at me as if I'd come from Mars. I interpreted his look to be saying, "What's this little kid doing, trying to tell us something?" And that immediately turned me off. The result was that I remained an ordinary student and failed to prepare and analyze my cases so I'd be able to handle questions. The results: Poor teaching leads to poor education. I resolved not to act that way when I was in a teaching situation myself, but vowed to emulate David Cheever and Castle. There is a special obligation one carries with him, as I do now sixty years after graduation, resulting from that August afternoon with George Minot. When I'm busy or too tired or lazy to take a dietary history, I think of George Minot. If he can take his time to teach me, just another face in the crowd, why can't I do the same?

Samuel A. Levine, an inspiring teacher with numerous gimmicks, was exposing our group of six to the rudiments of electrocardiography. One of us asked him, "Dr. Levine, if you could pick just one characteristic for the good physician, just one, what would you pick?" His response was immediate, "Generosity." He was referring not just to generosity with the purse, but with time, with colleagues, with persons up and down the socioeconomic scale, recognizing them as people. When Sir James Paget, the brilliant English surgeon-pathologist of the late 1800's, came on the wards, the first ones he addressed were the charwomen and this when British society was severely restricted by social class.

My third and fourth year surgery at the Peter Brent Brigham was heavily influenced by the professional and personal character of the resident staff because of their concern for patients, their interest in students, their striving for improvement of their scientific knowledge and technical skill. J. Englebert Dunphy went on to be chairman at San Francisco. Robert Gross was always meticulously dressed. He had beautiful hands and took blood painlessly from me using the large number fifteen needle. These men were undoubtedly influenced by the chief, Elliot Cutler. We all know the chief sets the standards on the service. The residents and interns, no matter how late they had been up the night before, were immaculately dressed in the morning, always shaved, their shoes whiter than white. They did not roam the wards in scrub suits. I have a picture of myself when I was the resident surgeon at New Haven: I am in a totally white outfit including necktie. I was so compulsive about neckties that when I was medical director of the Frontier Nursing Service in 1975, a couple of young physicians and several nurses rode up to my house on motorcycles at Christmas all wearing neckties over sweaters or overcoats or jackets. Patients expect you to look like their idea of a physician.

When I contracted the deadly Pneumococcus Type III pneumonia in my senior year at college, serum for other types of pneumonia was available, but not for mine. Everyone thought I was going to die. I don't remember waging a battle for my life. I simply wanted to roll over and withdraw. Yet, I still looked forward with anticipation to the visit of my physician, Dr. Harry French. He was there to see me every day and that had a profound effect on my recovery. When I became a doctor and had patients of my own, I saw them every day that I possibly could. I continued to do that at SSTAR in my work with drug addicts and alcoholics. I visited them every day: Saturday, Sunday, Thanksgiving or New Year's, because I hoped that my presence made a difference to them, as Dr. French's presence did for me.

The daily visit is especially important in a surgical career. Every now and then there is a subtle change in the patient's condition that indicates an approaching disaster if not warded off. If you see the patient daily you will detect trouble when you do his dressing, feel his pulse, or check with the nurse. Major trouble on Monday or Tuesday might have been avoided if you had been there on Sunday or New Year's and detected a small signal of impending complication. In surgery no one but the operating surgeon knows where the weak points of his procedure are. You know what to look for and what to expect. No other person is able to know this or have the information that will allow you to detect an early complication. You know about a suture line under too much tension or a bowel that didn't look that good or perhaps a tie you put on that might have been too tight or too loose. From my own illness, I learned always to warn my patients when I was about to hurt them. During my pneumonia episode, I, the college boy, was unnerved by a beautiful creature who said, "Mr. Lepreau, I'm not going to hurt you." She held my hand and, wham, a stilette hit my finger so she could do a blood count. I have never forgotten that double-cross. I learned about the seriousness of illness, especially in the elderly where recuperation is prolonged. Even at the age of 21, I spent two months convalescing.

In medical school, I roomed with three other students in the Boston Psychopathic Hospital where we did the laboratory work in return for room, board and laundry. One of our avocations was reading the old clinical pathological conferences from the Massachusetts General Hospital, called Cabot Cases, started by the famous Richard Cabot who had started the social service department of the Massachusetts General Hospital, the first of its kind. Cabot repeatedly disregarded laboratory findings and returned to the history and physical examination of the patient. I have continued the Cabot philosophy. It has made me think, made me analyze tests and has undoubtedly saved the system money. Also at Boston Psychopathic Hospital, Dr. Myrtle Canavan, the meticulous neuropathologist for the Commonwealth of Massachusetts, was a gentle lady who taught me kindness in a scientific way, and respect for a cadaver.

A year in pathology under Dr. Ralph Miller at the Dartmouth Medical School taught me not to cover up, not to be timid in pointing out the mistakes of others, but to do it gently. Next year, as a rotating intern I fell under the spell of various attending physicians, particularly Sven Gunderson, a Harvard Medical School product, not just because he was good medical mentor, but because he was gentle and kind to patients. The ophthalmologist John Coyle had the same gentleness. There were many other men at the Mary Hitchcock Hospital in Hanover, New Hampshire, from whom I learned the best medicine and science. The dour Dawson Tyson was my surgical ideal, a masterful technician imbued with the Halsted tradition learned at Johns Hopkins and Yale. He was responsible for my appointment to the surgical house staff at the Yale-New Haven Hospital where I progressed through the ranks to become the resident surgeon.

At New Haven, Max Taffel was an outstanding neurosurgeon, board certified in neurosurgery and thoracic surgery. Taffel was a great teacher and we all loved him even though he hardly ever let us tie a knot because of his commitment to the patient. "This patient asked me to do his surgery," he would say, "I'm obligated to do it." Later when I had residents who were reasonably competent, I allowed them to do perhaps half of my surgery, but I was always there from beginning to end.

In New Haven, when Dr. Lindskog was driving hard to get the chairmanship of surgery, he could be devastatingly caustic while running meetings. On the other hand, we all learned. One of my friends, who was an assistant resident with me, had a bad outcome with a patient. Lindskog looked straight at him and using his last name said, "K, you killed this man." This again brings up the question of who is the best teacher, the one who rubs you hard like that, or the one who is kind and gentle. Who knows? Each one has his own technique. We all knew Dr. Robert Zollinger's abrasive but fair technique. I spent considerable time with him as a student when he was attending at the Brigham. Although he polished me off several times, I really liked him. He taught me a lot.

There are numerous considerations about patient care but I'll just mention a few. My wife and I had a small green house where we grew camellias and I had planted a rose garden on our property. When they were in bloom I'd pick a blossom on the way out of the house in the morning and bring it to a patient. I liked to do it and the patient just thought it was great. Their doctor, especially a surgeon, was thinking of them. Also, in considering patient care, I always thought that a patient who had no appetite, but otherwise was doing well, would respond better if I could present him with some kind of food he liked. So I kept some expensive and usually nutritious food in the hospital refrigerator, perhaps a beef tenderloin or porterhouse steak, that I could order up from the kitchen. If they wanted something ridiculous such as marshmallows or shrimp, I would get that, too.

What is the future for physicians? I worry that my successors will be forced to sell themselves down the river like slaves to a corporation who will tell them what they can and cannot do, who will set their fees, causing them to end up just like so many other Americans, employees worried about a pink slip because they don't conform. Corporations are formed for service and profits, mostly profits. Corporations have stockholders. My successors' lives may be determined by those investors. This is anathema.   I don't think I could be a physician under such a system.   Perhaps the answer is single-payer government medicine.

What is the future of surgery? Operations of today will be extinct. Polio vaccine resulted in a sea change in orthopedics; no longer are teaching hospitals and Shriners Hospitals filled with reconstructive surgery due to that once mysterious malady. Surgeons rarely drain pus. Angiogenesis and angiostatin may one day alter the entire treatment of cancer. Today the devastating chemotherapy reminds me of erstwhile surgical infections, a scratch turned into an amputation or worse before antibiotics.   Fifty years hence students will ask, "Didn't they know any better?" No, we didn't. Perhaps surgery will be in congenital defects, trauma and organ transplantation.

Surgeons must continue to learn basic surgical principles and technique, be compassionate, exhibit sound judgment, and accept personal responsibility for the patient from the first incision to the final outcome.

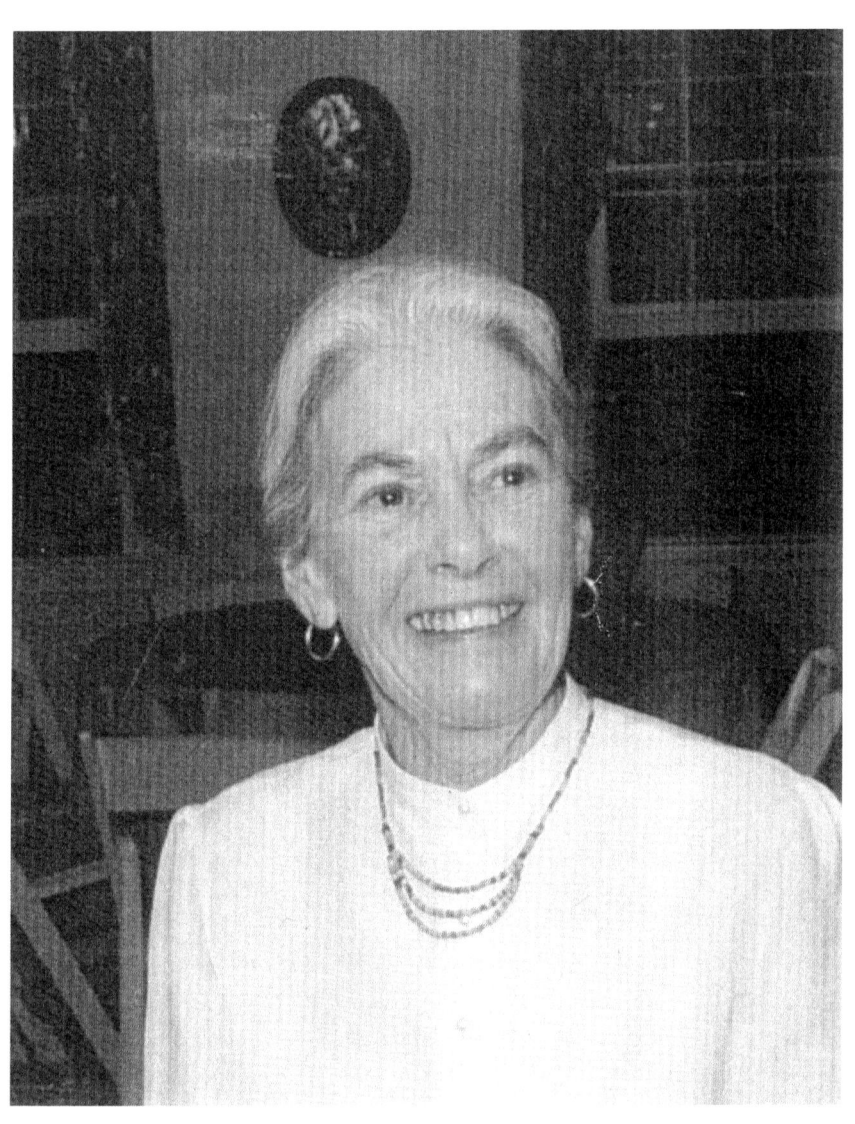

Wellesley Reunion

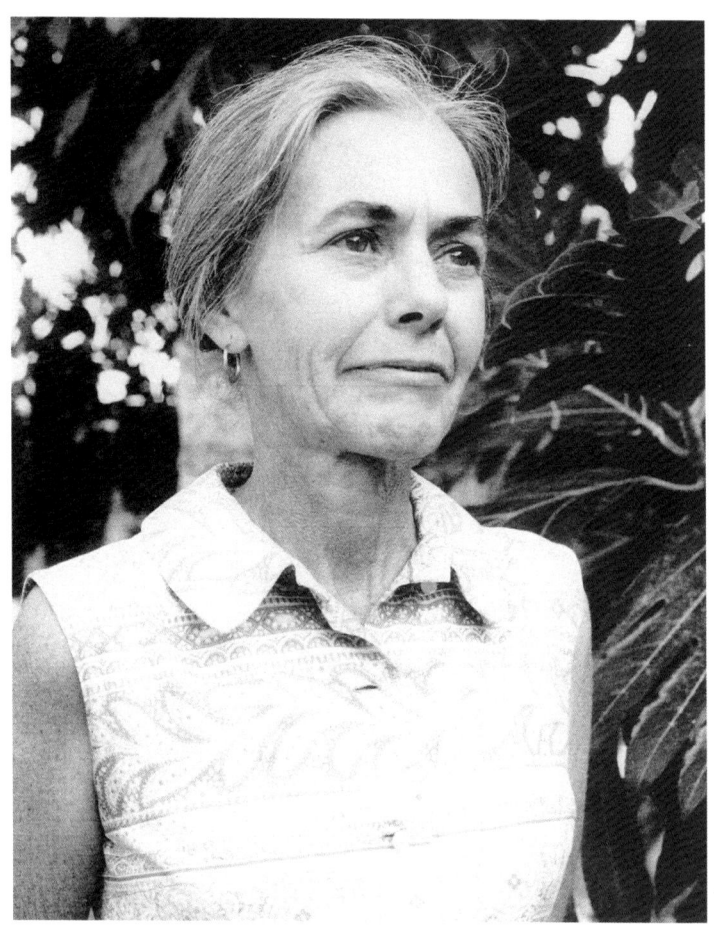

Monny - Talent Galore

13

A Love Story

I can recall the day and moment when I first met my wife, Miriam Barwood, as well as the final hours of our life together. What transpired in between was a lifetime rich with shared living and loving. Monny was my life. I cannot imagine having lived without her. But, back to the beginning. It was 1938, and I was in Hanover, New Hampshire, at my first position following graduation from medical school.

She walked into the small room where I was looking down a microscope at tissue slides and asked, "Is Dr. Miller in?" I turned and there she was, absolutely stunning in a snug tan sweater, plain reddish maroon wool skirt and brown and white saddle shoes, the standard equipment for a new college graduate. Dr. Ralph Miller was the head of the pathology department at the Dartmouth Medical School and Monny was seeking admission to his laboratory technician school at the nearby Mary Hitchcock Memorial Hospital in Hanover, New Hampshire. She had graduated in June from Wellesley and had returned to her family's home in Hanover to get a self-directed post-graduate course in music and "culture." Now, in September, her mother said, "Miriam, either you get out of the house or I will." She entered the technician school and rapidly became the best in the laboratory. Upon graduation she was assigned to a small cottage hospital in Littleton, New Hampshire.

After our brief conversation at that first meeting, I followed this Miss Barwood to the stairway, and then watched out the window as she drove off in a maroon Oldsmobile convertible. Lightning had struck. I told my fellow interns and residents in the laboratory to stay away. "She's mine!" She forgot the incident, but after she began working in the hospital laboratory where I occasionally appeared, she began to ask associates, "Who is this Dr. Lepreau?" I, too, was new, graduating that same June 1938 from Harvard Medical School. Chance encounters followed. I was the typical suitor, a little hesitant, yet persistent at the same time. Later that fall we both turned up at a square dance at the White Church in Hanover. There she was again, beautiful, petite, in a rust colored dirndl dress with embroidery. We danced and danced and danced and fell in love.

It was my habit to ride a bicycle from Dr. Miller's house to the hospital. I was broke and he had given me a room in his attic and a bicycle. Soon I began to take the long way around so I could pass the Barwood house for a glimpse of Monny or an occasional breakfast. We enjoyed late evenings, too, made even later by Mrs. Barwood's midnight donuts after her husband returned from Lebanon where he delivered the movies from the last show.

For Thanksgiving we went to the family ancestral home of Harty Beardsley, a friend from Dartmouth days. His mother, whose maiden name was Hartness, united two old New England names. Thanksgiving in the old stone house was right out of Dickens: big flaming logs in the fireplace, popcorn, dunking for apples and all the traditional trappings. When Miss Barwood and Dr. Lepreau walked from the car into the house, she said, "I suppose when we go in we should start calling each other by our first names." This was at Thanksgiving. We had met early in September.

One frigid winter night I pulled up at 6 Pleasant Street in a one horse sleigh, picked her up, silk stockings and all, freezing all the way over the Connecticut River to Norwich and back, but no ears, fingers or toes frozen! What love will do! In pursuit of Christmas presents we took a ridiculous trip to Vergennes, Vermont at night in a heavy snowstorm. We found and bought the prized wooden bowls, which were the excuse for the trip, got lost on the way home and, while attempting to turn around on an icy slope, slid within ten feet of Lake Champlain. Just before Christmas the laboratory at the medical school had a boisterous and liquid party. They drove me to White River Junction for the train to New York and home. Before boarding the train I called her from the station to express my undying love. But her pleasure turned to annoyance when she learned that my friends had pinned a note on my coat that said: "Throw me off at Hastings on the Hudson." New Year's was also spoiled for her when she was taking me to a party of her friends in a cabin in the woods. I drove the Oldsmobile into a ditch on an icy country road – broken axle. "Hello, Mr. Barwood".

Fortunately, Monny's father, Arthur Barwood, was easygoing. He was of medium height and bald and had been quite an athlete in his youth. He had been the golf champion of the Hanover Country Club twice, two years in a row. He managed the Nugget movie theatre. To finance his children's education he started additional businesses, letting them go when no longer needed. He had a tire retreading operation to get one child through, then a film transportation business, transporting movie films all over northern New England. He often took the film from the last show of the evening down to White River Junction, returning around midnight. Mrs. Barwood usually had donuts and coffee ready for him, which I occasionally shared. He bought a restaurant called Lou's and ran that for a while. He never lost money on these, but when the need was no longer there, he spent his time golfing and fly-fishing, at which he excelled. His wife, Edith, was a scrawny lady, somewhat hard of hearing, and always had a cigarette in her mouth. She was always good to me. Once Monny and I were smooching in the living room when I heard a cry from upstairs. "Frank, are you going to stay all night?" I scrambled up and started to tear out of the house. But she said, "No, I just wanted to know if you were going to stay all night. I can make up a bed for you in the backroom."

I met several of Monny's friends at a New Year's Eve event where we went to join them in a cabin somewhere in the beyond, the same night that I wrecked her father's car. Her husky friends got us out with their muscles, chains and a pick-up truck. Here again is an example of Monny's character. She never explained or apologized or made any remark about her personal friends who were somewhere down the socioeconomic scale from the faculty youth in Hanover. She was a townie. There was a social schism between faculty children and townies. She never made much out of it because it meant nothing to her. The former sent their children out of town to private schools. The townies went to the local public schools where Monny became the class valedictorian. Her independence was manifest in this and many other areas.

After Monny and I became engaged, her New Hampshire relatives were invited to meet me. But disaster loomed and was averted at the last moment. Dr. Miller and I were bringing his new Friendship sloop from Harpswell, Maine, to Falmouth Foreside. The boat trip was great, sailing on a starlit night with lots of colorful aids to navigation. But it was a long drive across Maine to the Barwoods and the family gathering. I made it just in time, but Monny was not happy.

Right from the beginning in 1939, when we were married, Monny was supportive of my career and showed it with her early gifts of medical books: Cushing's biography of William Osler, a biography of Hugh Hampton Young, the pioneer American urologist at John's Hopkins and many others. It is impossible to put into words her integrity, her intellectual brilliance, her physical beauty, ease and friendship with anyone, attention to the Lares and Penates of her household, and above all her unconditional devotion to her family. How I wish I could talk to her, as I often did while sitting in our old rocking chair and watching her on the sofa, her thin pink shawl around her shoulders, her hands busy with her knitting.

Writing up these lines reminds me again how fortunate I am that she gave her life to me. Monny was not all that excited to work at Hôpital Albert Schweitzer, particularly in the boring record room coding all the outpatient hospital diagnoses. She spent many hours a day, which was very helpful to the public health folks. She scrubbed with me on the chest cases. As instrument nurse she had a long table with many different tools

whose myriad names she learned rapidly. We became a
great team and worked harmoniously.

The remodeling of the house on Old Harbor Road
in Westport, where we finally settled after returning to
the States, worked out perfectly for her. She designed
her ideal kitchen, which took up the southeast corner of
the first floor. Kendrick Snyder ably executed it for her.
Here she had bright sun and a beautiful view of the yard
stretching away to the river. Above the kitchen on the
second floor was her sewing room where she worked at
the same machine that she had received from her mother
as a wedding present. I occasionally went in to see her
and to kiss her. She looked up at me with a mouth full of
pins that she quickly removed when she noticed my
intent.

This poem, "Nota Bene," by Helena O'Neill,
could have been written by Monny to me:

I will not mind if you forget
The way I used to smile,
The clothes I wore, the songs I sang,
My literary style.

The books I liked, the way I danced,
My thoughts, my shy demands,
My silly fears, my swift delights,
My perishable hands.

In future years you may forget
My eyes were granite blue,
But all your life and afterwards
Remember: "I loved you."

Monny was beautiful, elegant in dress and demeanor, always her own person, uninfluenced by others or social pressure. Solid integrity she had, and modest about her extraordinary intellect. Her raison d'etre was her family and we knew it. She was like the perhaps now obsolete construct of the atom. She was the nucleus about which we, the neutrons, were kept in proper orbit, held there by her love and character, not flying off into foolish or dangerous ventures. She was the ultimate role model. Even today I frequently ask myself, "What would Monny do?" I can never live up to her integrity or her devotion to her children and to me. But I do try. I try to make difficult decisions more promptly, as she did. Keep clean and neat at all times, avoid showing off. The more I can be like Monny, the better man I will be.

The last time I kissed Monny was when she was waiting for the fateful bronchial biopsy that began her demise. I wanted to kiss her despite the thrush throughout her mouth. Touching her forehead, she said, "Kiss me right here." These were the last words I heard from her as I kissed her for the last time. She spent the remaining days with an endotracheal tube on a ventilator: disaster and tragedy. She died undiagnosed and therefore we were reluctant to pull the tube, hoping for a miracle. The autopsy showed multiple pulmonary emboli, which could have been dissolved with medication then available. She also had a nest of cancer cells in the lymph nodes in both the right and left chest.

Her death was a failure of the art of medicine and I was part of the failure to put the pieces together, in short to make the diagnosis of treatable multiple pulmonary emboli, a condition well known to me and the attending physician. She had a successful left pneumonectomy by Dr. Alceu Pedreira, a skilled thoracic surgeon, partially trained by me, and a graduate from one of the best cardiothoracic residencies in the country. She had been maintained on coumadin for a few years because of cardiac auricular fibrillation. In recent months, preoperatively, parts of her visual field occasionally had obliterated, but she rapidly recovered. At surgery and in recovery she was maintained on what we thought was proper anti-coagulation. The proper diagnosis was finally considered and a bronchoscopy biopsy attempted to confirm it. She bled during the bronchoscopy without biopsy. The stage was set, even without the biopsy, but none of us put it all together, and she died of a treatable condition. Perhaps our failure prevented many months of a debilitating stroke or a painful wasting due to extensive cancer.

Monny's dying on a respirator was the final tragedy. Our only communication was the feeble and usually illegible notes she attempted. It was an inhuman, impersonal disaster for all. After sharing 54 years of wonderful closeness, we were now separated by a cold mechanical device that forbade oral communication because of the tracheal tube. She tried to write to me, but her hand had become too weak. Her small but clear penmanship had degenerated into an illegible scrawl. What was she trying to tell me? Knowing her, it was likely, "I love you" or "Take good care of the children." Fortunate we were that she gave her life to our family. Monny left us on June 2, 1994, with Jay beside her.

These verses from the last chapter of Proverbs could have been written of Monny:

Who can find a virtuous woman?
For her price is far above rubies.
The heart of her husband doth safely trust in her,
so that he shall have no need of spoil.
She will do him good and not evil all the days of her life.
She seeketh wool, and flax,
and worketh willingly with her hands.
She riseth also while it is yet night,
and giveth meat to her household,
and a portion to her maidens.
She layeth her hands to the spindle,
and her hands hold the distaff.
She is not afraid of the snow for her household:
for all her household are clothed with scarlet.
She maketh herself coverings of tapestry;
her clothing is silk and purple.
Strength and honour are her clothing;
and she shall rejoice in time to come.
She openeth her mouth with wisdom;
and in her tongue is the law of kindness.
She looketh well to the ways of her household,
and eateth not the bread of idleness.
Her children arise up, and call her blessed;
her husband also, and he praiseth her.
Many daughters have done virtuously,
but thou excellest them all.
Give her of the fruit of her hands;
and let her own works praise her in the gates.

14

Some Memorable Patients

Stone

I was an assistant resident in urology in the Yale-New Haven Hospital in 1941 when a lean, healthy forty-year-old male came into the clinic complaining of urinary frequency. The physical examination was negative. There were red cells in the urine. A plain film of the abdomen in preparation for a kidney study showed a huge bladder stone. Because he came through the clinic, he was "my case". I made the required incision in the abdomen and the bladder but neither my assistant nor I could get it out. Too big. Our hands could not get around it and it did not seem appropriate to break it up with a hammer. I said, "Send someone down from the obstetrical ward with obstetrical forceps." We delivered a two and a half pound stone with those forceps. But even so it was difficult to get out. In some parts of the world, notably India, large stones are common but none in the literature equaled our monster, which I reported in the *New England Journal of Medicine* in 1943.

Johnny

Johnny was twelve and helping out his father, an auto mechanic, when he was severely burned by an explosion of gasoline-soaked cloths stored in a large metal drum. As junior on the staff I was covering the emergency room at the Truesdale Hospital when he was brought in. His clothes had caught on fire and the burns involved chiefly the trunk and his legs. I can't remember a percentage. I had experience at the Hartford Circus fire and at New Haven doing considerable plastic surgery. Time was the most important consideration in an extensive burn case and I had plenty on my hands as I had just started to get patients. Most conscientious practitioners these days would send a badly burned patient to a burn center such as the Shriners Unit in Boston, but at that that time I don't think the unit had been built.

Taking care of Johnny required considerable fortitude on his part, lots of consoling and patience by the nursing staff and me. Eventually the secondary burns healed and then we worked on the grafting. It was a long course of at least two months but everything healed well and everyone was happy. As a result of that, I became the local burn expert and several other less demanding patients appeared until I inherited a much more challenging burn victim.

Johnny became a grateful patient. His buddy lived across the road on a farm. One evening these two young teenagers took me to Westport Harbor where we caught herring at the Herring Run Brook.

Burned

MJ was a ten-year-old boy who was at home after being hospitalized for extensive third degree burns. The old, open burns presented a horrendous challenge. The town nurse found him at home. She knew about my care of Johnny, so she asked me to visit him to see if I could do anything for him. MJ was a disheartening sight. He was curled up on a cot. His family was at a total loss about what to do. I got him to the Truesdale Hospital and a long, three-month saga began: painful dressings, improved nutrition, intravenous fluids and weekly skin grafting. I was now a busy practitioner. To avoid postponing MJ because of other patients who needed surgery, I designated Tuesday as MJ day. Each Tuesday we would do something for him—a skin graft or perhaps a major dressing. It was a technical challenge to get enough skin because he had few areas that were intact. Most often we took skin from his lower legs and had to recut the donor sites several times. This meant that each graft had to be very thin, yet thick enough to take and be reasonably durable. In order to minimize anesthesia problems we took him to the operating room and had everything all set up and organized, even draping him before the anesthesia was administered. It was used only for the actual cutting of the grafts which I laid on and held in place with a stitch here and there.

Eventually we got him all covered. The final result was a major accomplishment on the part of the patient to withstand the innumerable procedures and the nursing care. Fortunately I had the required technical ability.

I saw *MJ* sometime later and learned that he was managing satisfactorily. If his injury had occurred now, he would have been sent directly to the Shriners Hospital in Boston. *MJ's* family had no medical insurance. The surgical procedures, skin grafting and nutritional needs were horrendous. It was free treatment on my part and a big hospital expense, but dollars didn't figure into the case.

Why?

Ms. J, developed acute pancreatitis. This was a rare and disastrous complication that developed after I had performed a good sub-total gastrectomy for a duodenal ulcer, which was the standard treatment at the time when medical management failed. I had reoperated on her to see what I could do. It appeared that nothing could be done. Things seemed hopeless. I asked Dr. J. Englebert Dunphy, one of the country's best surgeons, from the Peter Brent Brigham Hospital to see her in consultation. Bert was a good friend. He was several years ahead of me at the Harvard Medical School and had been the resident surgeon at the Brigham when I was a student there. He came down on a Sunday morning with his wife. He recognized the magnitude of the problem and said, "Frank, you know we have a good house staff. We would be glad to take her off your hands." Why I refused his offer I cannot recall. For whatever reason, it was a colossal mistake. Bert and his group might not have saved her, but certainly would have relieved my tormented mind.

Patience

On another occasion, Dr. Dunphy helped my good friend, Edgar Cyr, and me with a happier outcome. Here I was hampered by a close friendship with a patient where my emotions threatened to overrule rational judgment. Edgar had regional enteritis, which is a chronic condition with ups and downs due to persistent inflammation of the small bowel. It sometimes caused obstruction. He was forty years old and in good shape. Nearly everyone in Fall River knew the happy, generous Edgar Cyr who ran his specialty food store on South Main Street. His counter girls made the best sandwiches in town and served the best coffee. The aroma of freshly ground and brewed coffee filled the atmosphere of his long, narrow shop, filled with all kinds of wonderful foods. You could put your hand in the barrel and pull out whatever you wanted.

But the time came when he had to be admitted to Truesdale under my care because the occasional abdominal pains had become severe, due to small bowel obstruction. After several days of observation and various stomach, intestinal and rectal tubes, he had not improved. Operation would be the easiest way out. I could cut the adhesions or untwist the bowel. But both Edgar and I knew that, although he would be immediately relieved, he could be left with more adhesions which would invite another episode of obstruction.

What to do? To cut or not to cut? Of course Edgar's health was my primary concern. So I again asked Dr. Dunphy to help me out, to help me decide what to do. He was nice to come down again. He interviewed and examined Edgar and studied the chart and the x-rays. We all gathered in Edgar's room No. 205 opposite the nurses' station on Charlton Two. Dunphy then suggested that I wait it out, and explained that during World War II, he had made rounds with the distinguished British surgeon, Sir Heneage Ogilvie. When they discussed a patient with a condition similar to Cyr's, Sir Ogilvie had said to Dunphy, "He will open up. Sounds that would make a duchess blush are music to the surgeon's ears". In a few days Edgar made those sounds, no blushing, but immense relief all around.

Patent Ductus

In 1951 in Fall River, I divided the patent ductus of a sixteen-year-old boy. This was the first for me and for Fall River. Fifty years later, in October of 2001, I met him once again. He is quite healthy, having survived two coronary artery by-pass operations. I performed about five or six patent ductus operations without problems. The only one that I ligated was in an adult. It cut through and endocarditis developed in the area, all of which was remedied by Dr. Robert Gross at the Boston Children's Hospital. I watched this very dangerous procedure. Dr. Gross did it with bravado and consummate skill.

Scalpel

One Sunday morning I was in the Truesdale Hospital early because my family had planned an excursion. As I entered the emergency entrance I heard a loud wheeze. It was not just an ordinary wheeze. There was something plaintive about it. It came from a middle-aged woman struggling for air. She bore a typical thyroidectomy scar on her neck, which a companion confirmed. He said she had trouble breathing ever since the operation but it became worse on damp or rainy days. We were fortunate to be where a scalpel was available. This was all I needed. For the first time in my life, I cut into her neck, into her trachea, rotated the blade and heard the life saving air rush in.

Disorders of the thyroid gland and its remedies were a challenging mystery when Caleb Parry, in 1780, first described what we now know as hyperthyroidism, over activity of the gland which causes extreme apprehension, nervousness, protruding eyeballs, exothalmos, tremor, sweating, loss of weight, all accompanied by a swelling in the anterior neck. In the early 1900's, it was realized there was an association between iodine and the thyroid. In areas like Switzerland where there was no contact with the ocean, people developed a large gland. Physicians knew they must get rid of the gland but the operation was frequently followed by a "thyroid storm." Thyroid storm is an exacerbation of all the basic symptoms of an overactive thyroid occurring during the immediate postoperative period. It was often fatal. Innumerable methods were devised to quiet the patient before surgery. Dr. George Crile at the Cleveland Clinic often did a mock operation in the patient's room. He brought the operating equipment and anesthesia machine to the bedside, put a mask on the patient's face, pretended he was going to perform the operation, and then he would leave. He might do this a couple of times, before the day he actually would operate. It was usually successful.

As a result of biological studies of marine life by others, Dr. Henry Plummer of the Mayo Clinic in 1922 recommended the use of ordinary iodine—ten drops in water, three times a day for ten days prior to the procedure. This changed the problem immensely. The operation could be completed, speed was no longer essential and the patient recovered well.

Theodore Kocher, a meticulous and sensitive Swiss surgeon, operated on many people who had enlarged thyroids. These people did not suffer from hyperthyroidism, just a huge gland. Many were young children or adolescents. There were no fatalities. He did a beautiful operation, but, much to his anguish, some ten years later these same children showed up as cretins, their growth stunted, and their metabolism low, pathetic blobs of humanity. They had become a cause of great anguish to this kind man because he had to face the fact that he was responsible. "I did it."

There were other complications of this procedure. After it was completed, the patient sometimes couldn't breathe well and the quality of the voice might change. If one looked down the larynx one could see that one or both vocal chords were paralyzed. A tiny nerve a bit smaller than the lead of a pencil enervates the chords. This nerve lies close to the back of the thyroid. The surgeon must be careful in his dissection to avoid injury. I have never injured one. In the meticulous surgery done by men like Kocher, this nerve was neither injured nor cut. In the modern era it is a technical, inexcusable error to cut both recurrent laryngeal nerves—as in my patient who was about to suffocate.

Other patients would occasionally go into tetany. Their muscles were hyperactive and would contract periodically causing a forced fixed smile. On tapping the facial nerve in front of the ear, the muscles of the face on that side would contract. This condition was caused by overly compulsive technical surgery. Along with the thyroid gland the surgeon removed two little glands on each side of the back of the thyroid which were the parathyroids controlling calcium metabolism. So, it is obvious that there were many facets in caring for thyroid diseases and until the early '40's, most of them involved surgery. Since then it has become almost a medical disease using radioactive iodine. Dr. Norman Hill at the Truesdale Clinic was the first person to use this technique in Fall River. It had to be carefully gauged so it didn't leave too many patients hypothyroid. There were drugs like Thiouracil, which suppressed the activity of the gland and probably others in the year 2004 of which I am not aware.

So there is a lot of history involved. I had a patient suffocating in the emergency room. She was overweight. She was probably hypothyroid because too much thyroid gland had been removed. The surgeon had not been careful and had cut, not one, but both laryngeal nerves. So she ended up with a distressing permanent tracheostomy and perhaps was required to take thyroid extract for the rest of her life.

Student Teaches the Teacher

One day at the Schweitzer Hospital in Haiti an infant appeared with a tracheoesophageal fistula, a fatal congenital anomaly, which we diagnosed promptly. The Yale resident with us had completed a rotation with Dr. Lawrence Pickett, a leader in pediatric surgery. I was an experienced thoracic surgeon, but had not done one of these difficult procedures in years. An Alphonse-Gaston Act ensued ending with my hands doing the operation, but Dr. Michael Curci talking me through it. Back in 1945, as the resident surgeon, I had taught Pickett, a fourth year student. And now 25 years later in the middle of that tortured land and thousands of miles from where we all learned, Curci taught Lepreau. The circle was closed. The patient did well.

Courage

Charlene Dondis is now alive and well. And, "I do remember it well." From Somerset, Massachusetts, she was eight years old when she came to the small and minimally equipped emergency room at Truesdale Hospital overlooking the Taunton River. Her foot had been run over and crushed by a truck, breaking the bones in her ankle and avulsing the full thickness of all the skin on her foot from her ankle to the toes. In fact, one toe was smashed. The wound was reasonably clean. I immediately took her to the operating room, cleansed the wound and completely covered it with the thickest skin I could cut from her back or buttock. I then set the broken bones and applied a cast. After a week I removed the cast and found that the graft was a complete take. The foot and leg were then immobilized for a month so that the bones would remain in good position and healing of the graft could be completed.

Now Charlene and her mother took over with appropriate physiotherapy and a follow-up with ballet lessons over many months. Charlene regained complete function and healing and I told them that the graft was perfect and would remain that way, but the sole of her foot would someday have to be replaced by a more durable full-thickness graft or pedicle graft of some type. *Mirable ductu*, almost fifty years later when I looked at it in March 2001 in Naples, Florida, I found she never needed it.

Yes, I did the proper original care and everything healed well. But her perfectly healed and functioning foot and leg was due to the courage of this young girl and to the persistence of her mother.

Wiring For Babies

The childless lady, whom I will call Madame Baptiste, came to Hôpital Albert Schweitzer because of frequent miscarriages. A barren Haitian woman, whether married or not, finds herself, not an outcast, but certainly not an acceptable spouse. Madame Baptiste became the first of a few people whom I successfully treated by circlage, which means circling the cervix of a pregnant woman with a wire—not difficult if one has a proper large needle with fused plastic-coated wire, which I did not have, but eventually acquired through the Yale residents. In the beginning I enclosed piano wire in intravenous tubing. The wire must be cut when the patient goes into labor or a ruptured uterus will result. To prevent such a catastrophe I found a nearby place where the lady could stay for the last month of pregnancy. I asked her to come to see me at least once or twice a week. I demanded that she wear the same orange patterned dress whenever she came to the clinic. I took her to every clinic and told each doctor that whenever she appeared in labor, day or night, to call me at once to cut the wire. It worked. We produced a few first babies and no disasters.

Father and Son

One Wednesday morning I had just finished my last case at Truesdale when a nurse came into the room. "Someone is calling you from Miami. He says he is a doctor," she said. It was *Dr. C.* He told me his father probably had tetanus (lockjaw), and no one in Miami knew how to treat him. "I am a thoracic surgeon like yourself." *Dr. C* said. "Would you be willing to come down and see him?" Of course I agreed and from that

point things went like a television serial: Off with my
gloves and gown, calls to the airlines in Boston and
Providence to get the first flight out of town, racing
through traffic to make my plane. On landing in Miami,
Dr. C met me at the gate and whisked me to his father's
bedside in an excellent Jewish hospital. He had scoured
the literature and found my name on two papers I had
written on tetanus. One cited my experience with more
than 600 cases in one year at Hôpital Albert Schweitzer in
Haiti.

I found the patient in total darkness in a quiet
room where the only light came from dials that
monitored pulse, blood pressure and respiration.   A
nurse sat beside him to regulate the intravenous carrying
the sedating medication. He was breathing comfortably
and was able to carry on a short conversation. His jaw
and all extremities were moderately stiff. I reviewed his
several medications, did a physical, studied the chart and
determined that he had a mild case of tetanus. If left
alone, except for small doses of diazepam to prevent
spasms, he would be fine. No need for darkness, no need
for other medications, and only fluids by mouth.
Everyone seemed happy, particularly his son who sensed
that I was confident of the diagnosis and the treatment,
and that he would survive. He did. *Dr. C* took me to a
sumptuous hotel room on the intercoastal waterway for
the night. It was bedecked with flowers and fruit. The
next morning the patient was stable and showing
improvement. I was put on the plane for Providence and
was soon back in Truesdale to make rounds. A twenty-

four hour ego trip, but I made everybody happy, particularly the son, whose zealous pursuit of the literature on behalf of his father had paid off.

How did this man get tetanus? He was a refugee from the concentration camps and had never been immunized. Recent dental work had stirred up the bacteria.

The Professor

The department chairman in a major medical center didn't feel well. He had no localizing complaints; he was just not his usual self. Nothing had been found in an extensive work-up in New York. He was now calling me in Westport to ask if I would check him over. Of course I would. A few days later when he appeared in my small Westport office, he looked his trim and alert self.

I was flattered that he thought a general and thoracic surgeon, now a family physician, could help him. I was under the gun, so I proceeded like a medical student interviewing a truck driver from Fall River. The past history, family history and the other details on a student's list yielded nothing. So I began the physical examination: head, eyes, ears, all the way down to the often neglected rectal. Bingo! He turned blue, had a chill, began to shake all over and became short of breath. I had made his diagnosis of chronic prostatitis. My digital examination had disturbed his prostate causing a shower of noxious bacteria to enter his blood stream. However I also had a major problem on my hands: a 60 year old man with a blood stream infection, having dyspnea, twenty miles from a hospital. I was frightened. Scared would be a better description. Of all people, my patient had to be my friend and one of the country's leading ophthalmologists, who had come up to me from New York to be fixed. Well, I was fixing him in a manner I did not like.

No catastrophe ensued. On the way to the hospital he improved. I took the usual blood and urine cultures, turned him over to my urologist, Dr. John Kaiser, who put him on intravenous antibiotics for a few days and sent him home on oral medications. He never had a recurrence. *Doctor L* was well known for his insight. He showed it by choosing a surgeon. We do rectals.

Mountain Man

I had not been back in Fall River very long before a nurse with whom I had worked years before asked me to see her husband for a second opinion. He was about to have a high amputation of his thigh, almost at the groin, because of a presumed malignant tumor. I thought it wise to at least try something less radical. Chris was a stocky woodsman type who camped and climbed in the White Mountains. Rugged he was. To lose a leg would be a disaster. Chris's original doctor was an orthopedist, so it fell to me to do the procedure. The tumor was huge, shaped like a watermelon and deep inside the muscular thigh. I successfully nucleated it without damage to vital structures or any cutting into this malignant leiomyosarcoma. We were lucky. There was complete healing and the man walked out of the hospital on the arm of his wife. He never had a recurrence. He had a garden and an orchard in nearby Assonet, and he kept me well supplied with fresh produce for years. And he returned to the mountains he loved for recreation.

15

Travels

In 1980, Monny and I went on a Sierra Club sailing jaunt in the South Pacific. I had just read Herman Melville's *Typee,* so I was anxious to experience the islands and tropical landscape firsthand. We flew to Hawaii, and then to the Marquesas, our first stop. From there we went on to Tonga where we spent several days. The British Royal family had recently honored their queen, Salote, who had died in 1965. In 1970 Tonga became a full partner in the British Commonwealth. We were privileged to spend time with Patricia Ledyard Mattieson who came there in 1949 to serve as headmistress of a girls' school. She met and married the local physician, a Scotsman. She has written two small paperbacks, *The Friendly Isles* and *Tonga Past,* which she gave to me. While there we visited the local markets and bought gifts made from the tapa cloth, woven from the bark of the mulberry tree.

In busy bustling Fiji we stayed at a large white edifice, the Grand Pacific Hotel, built in the waning empire days. Fiji is an example of who owns and operates the islands. The native Fijians are being crowded out by the more industrious Indians who control the economy much as in East Africa when I was there in 1961. While Monny was having a piece of coral removed from her leg at a public clinic, I was surprised to see a large bronze plaque hanging in the clinic foyer listing many British residents killed in WWII. We watched cricket players in their whites. We saw a replica, or maybe an original Fijian catamaran, which had a cabin-like enclosure and was used by the South Pacific islanders in their extensive exploration of the South Sea. We caught our first glimpse of American Samoa when we stopped at its only harbor, Pago Pago, a thoroughly westernized city. Tuna fishing was the chief source of income. Somerset Maugham's most famous story, "Rain", was so real in my mind that I felt cheated when no one could tell me where Sadie Thomson had lived. There was insufficient time to visit Western Somoa, an independent country. Robert Louis Stevenson's home, Vailima, sits on a hilltop with his grave nearby. The Mormons have recently rehabilitated his home and burial site. We found Mormon missionaries and an occasional physician on the smallest islands throughout the Pacific.

After returning from Haiti and settling in Westport, I had an opportunity to visit the Philippines. This resulted from my relationship with the Brown Medical School. Dr. David Greer, Dean of the school, asked me to visit the island of Leyte in order to assess an experiment in community-based medical education. Monny and Dr. Richard Olds went along, he to visit a schistosomiasis project. After a 22-hour flight to Manila we landed in a typhoon and were marooned in a hotel for three days. In Leyte the students start training as high school graduates and progress on a stepladder curriculum from nurse's aid to physician, combining their education with a paying position. The government hospital at Tacloban provided good clinical experience. I visited several classes. I recommended the program as an excellent way to keep medical practitioners in the semi-rural areas.

Exploring the area, I stood on Red Beach where my neighbor and friend, Bill Barker, as a GI, waded ashore under fire in the battle for Leyte Gulf, considered one of the great naval battles in history. Richard Hawes, another neighbor, was in one of our naval craft. I set out to visit Samar, a nearby island across a short bridge. The local advice was "You're crazy, but if you go, come right back." I could have been in danger of possible kidnapping by guerillas.

I made another Brown Medical School junket to the Caribbean to assess the St. Jude's Hospital in Vieux Fort, St. Lucia. Brown wanted to evaluate the facilities as a place for providing their students with "tropical medicine" experience. The hospital was well staffed and equipped, and because students and visiting physicians had been coming for years, it functioned like a teaching unit in an American hospital. A book called The Quest for the Killers by Jane Goodfield has a section called "The Three Valleys of St. Lucia" which describes clinical trials for the treatment of schistomiasis. We found no political problems in the area, there were beautiful beaches nearby and I recommended St. Jude's for our students.

~

In 1990, I was seventy-eight when I took a twelve-day trip on the Sandy, a 140-foot dragger, to George's Banks and back. Billy Tongue was the skipper. Earlier I had done some intricate and successful surgery on him. He was kind to take me along although in bad weather a person of my age could be a major detriment. The weather was good, the crew was kind, the food superb and I caused no problems except for my seasickness the first day out.

At about two and a half knots, the boat drags a huge net held down by rollers and heavy metal doors on the sides to keep it open. Periodically the net is pulled, the fish dumped on deck where the crew, with a three-foot pronged pole, sort out the yellow tail, haddock, cod and any other good fish and throw the rest overboard. The kept fish are immediately packed in layers of ice in the hold.

I made a contribution for my free ride: The bag is pulled up by a wire rope guided manually using a heavy iron bar to distribute the rope evenly along a horizontal spool. Suddenly the bar broke loose and hit the operator on the forehead causing a 10-centimeter laceration. I repaired it easily with steri-strips. I was a minor godsend, saving the time and gasoline that might have been used to return to New Bedford for medical help, and then return to sea. A few weeks later I learned that for several days afterward the patient had a runny nose. Obviously, as part of his scalp laceration he had broken the cribriform plate above his nose and he had a compound fracture of that part of his skull. The liquid from his runny nose was spinal fluid. He was most fortunate that he did not get meningitis.

When we returned to port in New Bedford we were held up overnight, I know not why. The merchants on shore set the prices for the catch and these can change rapidly, depending on supply and demand. If a skipper is delayed getting his catch to auction, the price could drop costing him considerable money and, because time is critical with fish, he must unload and sell at the going rate, whether he likes the price or not. The twelve-hour delay cost us money. But what is a skipper to do? You're right. He's stuck.

~

I had long wanted to see the Panama Canal. And so in 1995, I took a Caribbean cruise on an 85-passenger ship whose itinerary included the Canal. I was accompanied by Monny's best friend, Patience Barker Bryan, who was practically a member of our family. We went through the Canal by passing through a series of locks, which brought us up 85 feet from the Pacific and down to the Atlantic. We went from the Pacific Ocean over the Continental Divide through the Gatun Lake, which had been made by damming the Chagres River, and then down in steps to the Atlantic side, returning again to sea level. Alexander von Humboldt first suggested that the Atlantic and Pacific Oceans are at the same level when he explored South and Central America in 1799 to 1800. The huge lock doors functioned smoothly allowing for quick emptying and filling of the lock. We went through behind a container ship with its containers piled one on top of the other, five or six high. We were told that probably 48 ships had gone through the day we did, nearly a record. The canal was being widened and we saw steam shovels working as we went through the famous Culebra Cut, now called the Gaillard. Back in the 1900's the steam shovels were smaller than today's shovels, yet even these modern ones looked like teaspoons scooping away at the sides. George Washington Goethals was a senior engineer of the enterprise. Goethals' son was Professor of Obstetrics at Harvard Medical School and Number two at the Boston

Lying In Hospital and was one of my teachers there. I
don't know why, as I wasn't a good student, but the
doctor had an affection for me. I went out to his house
several times where we had Sunday lunch and listened to
Gilbert and Sullivan records.

Our narrator was John Mann, an American in his
late forties with pepper and salt hair and beard. He had
lived most of his life in Panama and was encyclopedic
about the history of the area, the Indians, the Darien
Jungle, and the San Blas Islands. He said the canal would
be widened with a combination of Japanese and
American contractors and engineers in concert with
Panama. Financing would come from international
shipping interests with the money passing through the
World Bank. The canal has considerable importance to
international transport, but of lessening importance to
the United States because of our transcontinental railroad
system with its mile long trains and cars often stacked
two containers high.

We visited the San Blas Archipelago, a chain of
365 islands scattered along the Caribbean coast of
Panama. The islands are close to sea level and are
protected by a long reef. Approximately 50 of them are
inhabited by the Kuna tribe and are heavily populated.
The people live in small flimsy buildings with minimal
support and I wondered how they survived tropical
storms. The soft-spoken people are small, broad of face,
with straight, black, shiny hair. The Kunas collect
coconuts and make and sell molas, squares of
multicolored appliquéd cloth, each one about 12 inches
square.

I spent time in the pilothouse with the captain
and watched him steer a fine line between several shoals,

drawing up to one of the beaches, which covered three or four acres. Once he was close enough, he dropped the ramp at the bow and we would walk ashore. Swimming in these warm tropical waters was perfect.

I enjoyed socializing with the passengers and listening to the various stories of their lives. Arthur was a good example and he proved to be a character. He is a short roundish man with a large, long cigar in his mouth most of the time. He has a contract to conserve energy at the Beth Israel Hospital, Lahey Clinic, Boston College, and another hospital, maybe the New England Medical Center. His overhead is minimal as he is the whole company. Mr. and Mrs. Justin Taylor, a couple in their mid sixties from Washington state, do extensive commercial shellfish farming and send the shellfish, mostly oysters, all over the United States. He is one of the main suppliers for Legal Sea Foods in Boston owned by the Berkowitz brothers. Taylor did 12 million dollars worth of business last year. There are many problems with organisms getting into the shells and with Indians who are about to lay claim to some of the islands. The Taylors and others like them, people with education, the ambition to do something and the will to make it happen, are a fascination to me.

~

I was eighty-five years old when I made a ten-day trip on a replica of the *Bounty*, the ship of the notorious Captain Bligh with its mutinous crew. It came about in February of 1997 when I visited my grandson, Peter Keller, who was a carpenter with the group in Fairhaven, Massachusetts restoring the 36-year-old boat that had been built for the movie, *Mutiny on the Bounty*, starring Marlon Brando. The boat was small, 120 feet long excluding the bowsprit, but still one third larger than the original. It was in poor shape and when it finally went to sea was not much better. I thought it would be fun to cadge a ride on her as she made her way down the coast, around the Florida Keys to St. Petersburg. After much talk and with the always helpful "carrying charges" of Sidney Greenstreet of *Casablanca*, the skipper agreed to pick me up in Charleston, South Carolina.

A few weeks later I was in Boston, ready to leave. Geraldine Kohlenberg Zetzel, the mother of my one-time lawyer, Max, joined me there for supper and the ballet, *Giselle*. She then drove me to Logan airport for a midnight flight to Charleston. Geraldine is a summer resident of Westport Point where I met her, a lovely Bryn Mawr graduate. Arriving in Charleston, I found that the airport was quite a distance from dockside where I was to pick up the Bounty. There were three passengers left on the plane and no one alive and well around the airport. How was I going to get to Charleston's docks? A pilot, who was on my flight as a passenger, helped me out with a ride to the docks. There I stood at four o'clock in the morning surrounded by black spars, hulls, hulks, docks, water and an eerie loneliness. I did not know where I was or where the *Bounty* was. I wandered around with my bag in my hand feeling foolish. Then with no sound or warning Peter suddenly appeared out of nowhere. I was glad to see him.

This *Bounty* expedition was probably unwise at my age, but I had a great time. The ship bounced around and I careened from side to side constantly holding on. If I had fallen and injured myself it would have been a

problem for my own health and a larger one for my
colleagues who would have had to get a helicopter to
evacuate me. But there were no falls or problems. We
sailed from Charleston around the Keys and up to St.
Petersburg. When we were fifteen miles from Cape
Canaveral we saw a space ship launched across the sky, a
spectacular cylinder of fire--white, yellow and red--like a
giant Roman candle. While off the coast at Miami we lost
all our lights including the red and green running lights.
It was cold as I stood my watch from midnight to 4 am. I
thought our situation a bit chancy as we were in the
smuggling area among speedboats, also with no lights.
The engine tired out so we did not have water, which
meant putting a bucket over the side for water to pour
into the johns. Finally we came into St. Petersburg,
pretty much intact. Throughout this risky adventure,
Peter was a great reassurance to his 85-year-old
landlubber grandfather.

16

Concluding Thoughts

In 1994 I began to serve as the Medical Director of the Rose Hawthorne Lathrop Home in Fall River, run by the Dominican Sisters of Hawthorne, whose corporate title is The Servants of Relief for Incurable Cancer. There were no gimmicks. We accepted patients from all over New England. From this experience I learned what we surgeons could do at the end of life.

Eliminate most of the innumerable medications our patients accumulate which are useless in their current situation. I stop most of them on admission. A terminal cancer patient needs pain relief, a tranquil mind, a night's sleep and a good bowel movement. Do not underestimate the importance of the bowels. One can learn about pain control without the use of needles from your local hospice.

Laboratory tests are not needed. What use is a blood ammonia in a patient with a large liver and palpable metastases? The hospital summaries accompanying the patient suggest Benjamin Rush at work. Your patient may need a transfusion to replace the blood drawn.

X-rays are equally unnecessary. Your scribbled "CT scan" on the order sheet initiates a long, unpleasant trip up and down elevators, through corridors, double doors and onto a hard table. Next the trip into a claustrophobic tube surrounded by scary, mysterious clicking noises. And it is always cold. The thin cotton blankets are never enough. All this to confirm what we already know. You suspect congestive heart failure? No need for chest films, EKG or echocardiogram. Just listen to the lungs, feel for the rate and rhythm of the heartbeat, and look at the ankles. Then give a little Lanoxin and Lasix and you are in business.

So what have we done? To satisfy our so-called intellectual curiosity, or to put together a Massachusetts General Hospital Clinical Pathological Conference, or to fend off a lawsuit, we have inflicted pain and mental anguish on a dying patient who has put his life and trust in "my doctor." Plain and simple, it is cruelty in the guise of scientific study.

Most important, do not abandon your patient. Without being too sentimental, there is a special bond between a patient and his surgeon. So in the final days when the chemo people, the chaplain, the radiologists, the social workers, the consultants, the myriad of do-gooders are constantly in and out, we must continue to visit daily to justify the trust the patient has given us.

~

What follows are excerpts from a speech I gave at a Brown University Medical School Graduation. I titled it *Being There*.

To a sick person there is no substitute for his healer, especially if the healer is someone known to him from personal association. Historically, witch doctors have taken the role of healer and under various guises they are alive and well today in such diverse places as Haitian lacours and even in Burlington, Vermont where some allergists I know rarely give injections.

In modern times, doctors of medicine are the healers, but only recently have they had any method of healing anyone. The medical men treated fevers with Jesuit bark from Peru, later identified as quinine. They rubbed mercury into the skin to treat syphilis; hence the old medical school saw, "One night with Venus, the rest of your life with Mercury." Withering's "An Account of the Foxglove," was not published until 1785. Surgeons cut for bladder stones, dressed wounds, amputated legs, and drained pus. Surgery was primitive until anesthesia was introduced in 1846 and antisepsis in 1867.

How was it, then, that the Jewish Maimonides, the French Rene Laennec, the English John Fothergill, and the American Benjamin Rush became the great physicians of their times? They cupped; they purged; they bled. Rush is said to have shed more blood than any general in history. They must have had something going for them if their patients survived such vigorous therapy and loved them.

Those medical ancestors of ours were effective because they were there—there with their patients, concerned and caring. Maimonides, when he had finished his official obligations to the Court of Saladin, returned to his lodgings, dead tired, to find patients waiting in the street and crowded together on his doorstep. He reassured them, tended their minor maladies, and educated them. Way back in 1190 he wrote in *The Aphorisms of Moshe*, "Most people get sick through too much eating and too little work."

Laennec, the scholarly clinician-pathologist, spent five years of his short life attending wounded Breton conscripts as they returned from the Napoleonic battlefields to the strange and frightening Paris hospitals.

Laennec was from Brittany and he was the only physician in the city who spoke their dialect. He could both dress the wounds and ease the minds of those rural people.

Fothergill made house calls and climbed stairs all over London. He not only described streptococcal sore throat, tic douloureux and angina pectoris, but he also provided a reassuring presence and support for the troubled spirit. Rush stayed behind to tend the sick in Philadelphia when thousands, including the city's physicians, fled during the yellow fever epidemics of the late 1700's.

Physicians underestimate the witch doctor's potential, the laying-on-of-hands effect. We get caught up in being au courant with the latest journal article or the upmanship we've made or heard at hospital rounds. How many times have we heard patients say, "Oh Doctor, I feel so much better when I see you." The effectiveness of Norman Vincent Peale's "power of positive thinking," the often-salutary influence of Christian Science, and the evil control exerted by Jim Jones attest to the power of the mind.

I am not suggesting that physicians take a course in hypnotism or humanism. I am suggesting that we take to heart the inscription on the statue of Edward Livingston Trudeau at the tuberculosis sanatorium he founded in the Adirondacks: "Cure sometimes, relieve often, comfort always." This inscription, at once humbling and challenging, acknowledges the ability we have to cure most infectious diseases and a fair number of surgical conditions, but also calls on our more demanding responsibility to give physical and mental support to those in the process of cure, to those we can only help, and to those whose pain and loneliness we can only assuage. If we are there, we will meet that demand; but we must be there, and that is the rub.

Being there takes time. Are we willing to take that time? Many doctors, younger than I, are intelligent, interested, conscientious, but protective of their time off. They take a lot of it, spending it with family and in athletic pursuits. It's hard to fault that behavior, but my generation wasn't geared that way and most of us had a good family. We made rounds on our days off, and we still do. Our home numbers were listed in the telephone book. If we are there beside our patient, we can easily relieve his mind with answers to questions that seem to him complex and mysterious. We can unblock the Levine tube to stop his vomiting. We can give the intravenous Lasix because we recognize that his slight cough is early pulmonary edema and not a cold, as the patient or nurse thought when we were called. We will recognize a subtle change in our patient's condition telling us that now is the time to operate, or that he's getting better and everyone can relax. We can see for ourselves whether the chemotherapy, the multiple operations, and the machinery are really helping, or if we have let them become refined cruelty under the guise of science. But such deductions can be made only by our careful observation, and we must be there to observe.

All this has a very personal meaning. When, as a college student, I was sick with pneumonia, I was under the care of a compassionate physician — quiet, reassuring and supportive. I could depend on my doctor's being there, and I learned so well how much that business of being there means to a sick person. The days of my illness were interminable, full of apprehension, loneliness and fear, alleviated only by the frequent visits of my doctor. His reassuring presence comforted and supported me while, at the same time, he silently observed and evaluated my condition. His visits kept him informed of slight but significant changes in my condition. And although, on occasion, Dr. French was only a blur of gray hair and a suit with a red tie, his vists always made me feel better.

Robert Louis Stevenson died of tuberculosis in Samoa at the age of 44. He had been attended by physicians in various parts of the world, and from a strictly scientific standpoint, they could do nothing for his malady. Stevenson wrote of his physician, "Generosity he has, such as is possible to those who practice an art, never to those who drive a trade: discretion, tested by a hundred secrets; tact tried in a thousand embarrassments, and what are more important, Herculean cheerfulness and courage."

Our profession remains an art. If we want to do our best for our patients and for our own tranquility, concentrate on the patients and then on learning. Eschew commerce. Don't get in a financial bind with too many encumbrances. Money problems are the single disease we physicians are not trained to fight; it can corrupt or destroy us.

What did *being there* mean to the people of Hôpital Albert Schweitzer? The model was set by the sign on the hospital at Lambarene in Gabon. "Here, at whatever hour you come, you will find light and help and human kindness." Larimer Mellon, Gwen Mellon and Walborg Petersen made it possible for us all to share in that experience.

The life of a surgeon is exhilarating, worrisome, and demanding--demanding of judgment, of dexterity and assumption of total responsibility for pre-operative decision-making, the operation itself, and recovery. Most bad outcomes are the result of technical or judgment errors. Tender, demonstrable compassion and scientific competence are required; either one alone is unacceptable.

Doctors in training are among the most fortunate in society. College and medical school and residency add up to twelve or thirteen years of an exciting learning experience, which is a reward in itself. Physicians are able to aid, frequently to cure, a suffering human being. A few of us will make discoveries advancing the healing powers of our ancient art. Who else has it so good? My professional career ended on August 15, 2002, six weeks short of my 90th birthday, when Rose Hawthorne closed. As Charlie Brown would say, "Not bad, not bad at all."

Surgery and Beyond

CURRICULUM VITAE

PERSONAL INFORMATION:

NAME: Frank James Lepreau, Jr., M.D.

DATE OF BIRTH: October 6, 1912

PLACE OF BIRTH: Oak Park, Illinois

CITIZENSHIP: United States

MARITAL STATUS: Widowed

HOME ADDRESS: 74 Old Harbor Road
                         Westport,
                         Massachusetts 02790

EDUCATION:

Undergraduate: Dartmouth College
                         Hanover, New Hampshire
                         B.A. Chemistry 1934

Medical School: Harvard Medical School
                         Boston, Massachusetts
                         M.D. 1938

POSTGRADUATE TRAINING:

Internship: Mary Hitchcock Hospital
                         Dartmouth Medical School
                         Hanover, New Hampshire
                                 Intern Pathology 1938-1939
                                 Rotating Intern 1939-1940

                         Yale-New Haven Hospital
                         New Haven, Connecticut
                                 Intern Surgery 1940-1942
                                 Asst. Resident, Surgery 1942-1944
                                 Resident Surgeon 1944-1945

PROFESSIONAL LICENSES AND CERTIFICATIONS:

State of Connecticut:	January 25, 1942
State of Kentucky:	May 29, 1974
State of Massachusetts	September 12, 1946
State of Rhode Island	1979
American Board of Surgery:	November 21, 1946
American Board of Thoracic Surgery:	April 14, 1950

ACADEMIC APPOINTMENTS:

Yale Medical School, New Haven, Connecticut
        Instructor, Surgery, 1945-1946
        Assistant Clinical Professor, Surgery, 1967 - 1975

Brown University Medical School, Providence, Rhode Island
  Assistant Clinical Professor of Surgery, 1979 - 1991
  Assistant Clinical Professor, Community Health, 1979 – 1991
  Assistant Clinical Professor, Community Health, Emeritus, 1991

HOSPITAL APPOINTMENTS:

Truesdale Hospital, Fall River, Massachusetts
        General and Thoracic Surgery, 1947 – 1964
        Chairman, Intern/Resident Committee, 1947 – 1964
        General and Thoracic Surgery, 1973 – 1974
        Director of Medical Education, 1973 – 1974

Frontier Nursing Service, Wendover, Kentucky
        Surgeon and Medical Director, 1974 – 1975

Westport Family Medicine Center, Inc., Westport, Massachusetts
        General Surgery and General Practice, 1975 – 1988

Charlton Memorial Hospital, Fall River, Massachusetts
        Chairman, Education Committee, 1976 – 1980
        Chairman, Department of General Surgery, 1981 – 1983

St. Anne's Hospital, Fall River, Massachusetts 1977 – 2002

OTHER APPOINTMENTS:

Hospital Albert Schweitzer, Haiti
        Medical Director, 1964 – 1973
        Surgeon, 1964 – 1970
        Chief of Surgery, 1970 – 1973
        Director, Grant Foundation, 1966 – 1973

Surgery and Beyond

Stanley Street Treatment and Resources, Inc., Fall River, Massachusetts
   Medical Director, Center for Alcohol and Drug Problems, 1977 – 1997
   Medical Director, Community Health Clinic, 1992 – 1997

Rose Hawthorne Home, Fall River, Massachusetts
   Medical Director, 1994 – 2002

Co-Founder of Fall River/New Bedford Center for Alcohol Problems, now Stanley Street Treatment and Resources, Inc., Fall River, Massachusetts

Co-Founder of Samaritans, Fall River, Massachusetts

Co-Founder of Hospice, Fall River, Massachusetts

Permanent Board, New England Yearly Meeting of Friends

Westport School Committee, Westport, Massachusetts
Lincoln School Committee, Providence, Rhode Island
Clerk: Monthly Meeting of Friends, Westport, Massachusetts

HONORS AND AWARDS:

B'Nai Brith, Man of the Year, 1961

Golden Deeds Award, Exchange Club, Fall River, Massachusetts, 1976

Honorary Doctor of Humane Letters, 1988, University of Massachusetts – Dartmouth

Nathan Smith Distinguished Service Award from the New England Surgical Society – 1996

Volunteer M.D. Award of the Year from the Massachusetts Medical Society – 1998

MEMBERSHIP IN SOCIETIES:

   American College of Surgeons
   New England Surgical Society, Vice President, 1977
   Massachusetts Medical Society
      Executive Committee, Past
      Blue Shield Committee, Past
      Impaired Physician Committee, 1979 to 2002

PUBLICATIONS:

Instrumental Removal of a Two-and-a-Half-Pound Bladder Calculus, with Recovery, Lepreau, F.J. and Jenkins, R.H., The New England Journal of Medicine, 229:25, P. 937, 1943.

Adult Tropical Intussusception in Haiti, Greco, R.S. and Lepreau, F.J., Archives of Surgery, 106:689-691, 1973.

Surgery in Haiti: Archives of Surgery, 107:483, 1973.

Ocular Manifestations of Xeroderma Pigmentosum in a Black Family, Bellows, R.A.,Lahav, M., Lepreau, F.J., Albert, D.M., Arch Ophthalmol, Yale University School of Medicine, 92:113-117, 1974.

Tetanus in Patients Three Years of Age and Up; 230 Consecutive Cases, (Dicussion by Lepreau, F.J.) Garnier, M.J., American Journal of Surgery, 129:459-463, 1975.

Tetanus in Haiti: THE LANCET, February 15, 1975, p.383 Garnier, M.J., Marshall, F.N., Davison, K.J., Lepreau, Jr., F.J., Departments of Anesthesia, Pediatrics and Surgery, Hospital Albert Schweitzer, Deschapelles, Haiti.

Low Anterior Resection of Colon and Anastomosis with Staples, Archives of Survery, 113:1479, 1978.

The Consultation: Archives of Surgery, 118, 1963.

Letters to the Editor, The New England Journal of Medicine:
        310: 13, 857, 1984 - Cost Effective Surgery
        312: 20, 1332, 1985 - Rationing of Medical Care
        315: 16, 1032, 1986 - Home Care, Who Cares
        322: 6, 406, 1990 - Adverse Outcomes and Lack of Health Insurance
        Among Newborns.
        330: 14, 1012, 1994 - Doctors and The Clinton Plan
        332: 20, 1386, 1995 - Foxglove
Obituary: William Larimer Mellon, Jr., M.D., J.A.M.A. 262:2391, 1989.

Community Based Medical Education in the Philippines, J.A.M.A., 263:1624-1625, 1990.

One Physician's Mission, Lepreau, F.J., Rhode Island Medical Journal, 74:179-182, 1991.